Unresolved problems in Haemophilia

Unresolved problems in Haemophilia

EDITED BY

Charles D. Forbes and Gordon D. O. Lowe,
University Department of Medicine
Royal Infirmary, Glasgow

*Proceedings of an international symposium held at
the Royal College of Physicians and Surgeons,
Glasgow, September 1980*

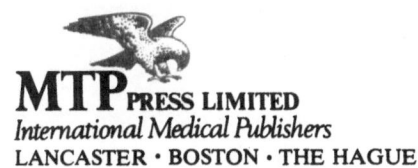

MTP **PRESS LIMITED**
International Medical Publishers
LANCASTER · BOSTON · THE HAGUE

Published in the UK and Europe by
MTP Press Limited
Falcon House
Lancaster, England

British Library Cataloguing in Publication Data

Unresolved problems in haemophilia.

1. Haemophilia – Congresses
I. Forbes, C.D.   II. Lowe, G.D.O.
616.1'572   RC642

ISBN 978-0-85200-388-6   ISBN 978-94-011-9764-9 (eBook)
DOI 10.1007/978-94-011-9764-9

Published in the USA by
MTP Press
A division of Kluwer Boston Inc
190 Old Derby Street
Hingham, MA 02043, USA

Library of Congress Cataloging in Publication Data

Unresolved problems in haemophilia

Includes bibliographical references and index.
1. Hemophilia-Congresses. I. Forbes, C. D.
(Charles Douglas), 1938- . II. Lowe, G. D. O. (Gor-
don Douglas Ogilvie), 1949- . [DNLM: 1. Hemophilia-
Congresses. WH 325 U61 1980]
RC642.U56   616.1'572   81-20754
                                       AACR2

Copyright © 1982 MTP Press Limited

Softcover reprint of the hardcover 1st edition 1982

Contents

Foreword

These proceedings are of a symposium held jointly by the UK Haemophilia Centre Directors and the Royal College of Physicians and Surgeons of Glasgow. The purpose of the meeting was to highlight the growing areas of haemophilia care and research as they serve as a model for the study of other disorders. In particular a major section of these proceedings is devoted to the investigation of liver disease in haemophilia – an area which offers unique opportunities for both basic, applied and clinical research. The second section considers modern treatment of bleeding disorders and the potential cost to society. With the advent of better standards of care, the requirements of plasma products have risen to such an extent that future predictions suggest a worldwide shortage may occur. The third section of the book discusses the detailed structure of the Factor VIII molecule and its sub-components and also its functional and immunological characteristics. The availability of amniocentesis and its accuracy in predicting which factor is affected has produced new problems for genetic counselling. The fourth section is clinical and describes the experience of procedures in the Nuffield Department of Orthopaedics, Oxford. For all of us looking after such patients this remains the most important unsolved clinical problem.

C.D. Forbes
G.D.O. Lowe

List of Contributors

Professor Charles Abildgaard,
Department of Paediatrics,
4301X Street,
Sacramento,
California   95817

Dr. L. Aledorf,
The Mount Sinai Medical Center,
The Mount Sinai Hospital,
1 Gustave L. Levy Place,
New York   NY 10029

Dr. M. Bamber,
Department of Medicine,
Royal Free Hospital,
Pond Street,
Hampstead,
London   NW3 2QG

Professor A.L. Bloom,
Professor of Haematology,
University Hospital of Wales,
Heath Park,
Cardiff

Dr. Colin Cameron,
Department of Virology,
Middlesex Hospital,
Mortimer Street,
London   W1P 7PN

Dr. John Craske,
P.H.L. Withington Hospital,
West Didsbury

Dr. Geijlswijk,
Department of Haematology,
University Hospital,
Utrecht,
The Netherlands

Professor John Graham,
Department of Pathology,
University of North Carolina,
Chapel Hill,
North Carolina,   U.S.A.

Professor H.C. Hemker,
Faculty of Medicine,
State University of Limburg,
Biomedical Centre,
Maastricht,
The Netherlands

Dr. Margaret Hilgartner,
Associate Professor of Pediatrics,
Director of Hemophilia Clinic,
Cornell University Medical Center,
525 East 68th Street,
New York   NY 10021

Mr. Gregory Houghton,
Nuffield Department of Orthopaedics,
Nuffield Orthopaedic Centre,
University of Oxford,
Headington,
Oxford   OX3 7LD

Dr. C.R. Howard,
Senior Lecturer,
Department of Medical Microbiology,
London School of Hygiene and
                    Tropical Medicine,
Keppel Street,
London   WC1E 7HT

Dr. Leon Hoyer,
Professor of Medicine,
Hematology Division,
University of Connecticut,
Health Centre,   School of Medicine,
Farmington,
Connecticut   06032

Dr. P.B.A. Kernoff,
Consultant Physician and Director
    of the Haemophilia Centre,
Royal Free Hospital,
Pond Street,
London   NW3 2QG

Dr. C.A. Ludlam,
Consultant Haematologist,
The Royal Infirmary of Edinburgh,
Lauriston Place,
Edinburgh

Professor R.N.M. MacSween,
Department of Pathology,
Western Infirmary,
Glasgow

Dr. R.S. Mibashan,
Department of Haematology,
King's College Hospital Medical School,
Denmark Hill,
London   SE5 8RX

Mrs. S. Middleton,
Blood Product Laboratory,
Elstree,
Herts

Dr. I.R. Peake,
Department of Haematology,
University Hospital of Wales,
Health Park,
Cardiff

Dr. F.E. Preston,
Consultant,
Department of Haematology,
Royal Hallamshire Hospital,
Sheffield

Dr. C.R. Rizza,
Oxford Haemophilia Centre,
Churchill Hospital,
Headington,
Oxford   OX3 7LJ

Dr. Chas. Rodek,
Consultant Obstetrician,
Kings College Hospital Medical School,
Denmark Hill,
London   SE5 8RX

Professor Peter J. Scheuer,
Department of Histopathology,
Royal Free Hospital,
Pond Street,
London   NW3 2QG

Dr. Howard Thomas,
Medical Unit,
Royal Free Hospital,
Pond Street,
London   NW3 2QG

Dr. David R. Triger,
Senior Lecturer,
Department of Medicine,
Royal Hallamshire Hospital,
Sheffield

Dr. J.G.E. Underwood,
Senior Lecturer,
Department of Pathology,
Royal Hallamshire Hospital,
Sheffield

Professor R.F.A. Zwaal,
Rijksuniversiteit Limburg,
Faculty of Medicine,
P.O. Box 616,
6200 MD Masstricht,
The Netherlands

SECTION 1 # Liver Disease in Haemophilia

Opening remarks

R. N. M. MacSween

Historically, you will recall that when Blumberg and his colleagues first discovered Australia antigen they used as their screening serum one derived from a multiple-transfused haemophilia patient from New York[1]. They were much intrigued as to why such a patient had developed a precipitating antibody in his serum which reacted with material present in the blood of an Australian aborigine[2]. Their subsequent investigations led to their demonstrating an association of this antigen with hepatitis[3], and from this single discovery in 1967 has stemmed our now very considerable knowledge of viral hepatitis. The association of Australia antigen was of course with serum hepatitis or hepatitis B, and the antigen is now known as hepatitis B surface antigen – HB_sAg.

It was anticipated that the screening of blood donors for HB_sAg would substantially reduce the incidence of post-transfusion hepatitis. However, this was not the course of events and, while some reduction did occur, post-transfusion hepatitis remained and remains a significant clinical hazard. It is now established that there are other transmissible agents capable of causing post-transfusion hepatitis, and there is good evidence that more than one virus is involved in what has become defined as non-A, non-B hepatitis.

Of particular interest has been the discovery that non-A, non-B hepatitis is a hazard in haemophilia patients and, as you will hear this afternoon, has been particularly associated with the use of the various concentrates with which these patients are now managed. Thus, while the use of these concentrates has represented a major advance in the therapy of haemophilia, it is unfortunate for the patients that this may be accompanied by an increased risk of acute and, possibly, chronic liver disease.

4

We are only at the beginning of investigation into the epidemiology of post-transfusion (or post-concentrate!) hepatitis in these patients. However, advances have already been made and some of the clinical, immunological and histological aspects of one type of non-A, non-B hepatitis have been documented in studies on haemophilia patients. It is a fair assumption that further progress in our understanding of hepatitis will derive from an extension of these studies. Thus, as with hepatitis B, the investigation of hepatitis non-A, non-B has received a significant stimulus from the haemophilia patient. It is indeed appropriate therefore, that at this meeting, devoted to unresolved problems in haemophilia, this first session deals with liver disease in these patients.

REFERENCES

1.   Blumberg, B.S., Alter, H.J. and Visnich, S. (1965).   A "new" antigen in leukaemia sera.   J. Am. Med. Assoc., 191, 541

2.   Blumberg, B.S. (1971).   Introduction and historical review. In: J.E. Prier and H. Friedman (eds) Australia Antigen, pp. 1 (London and Basingstoke: The Macmillan Press Ltd.)

3.   Blumberg, B.S., Gerstley, Betty Jane S., Hungerford, D.A., London, W.T. and Sutnick, A.I. (1967).   A serum antigen (Australia antigen) in Down's syndrome, leukaemia and hepatitis.   Ann. Intern. Med., 66, 924

1 The epidemiology of Factor VIII and IX associated hepatitis in the UK

Public Health Laboratory, Withington Hospital

Since 1969 the Oxford Haemophilia Centre on behalf of the UK Haemophilia Centre Directors has collected information about the incidence of jaundice after transfusion of Factor VIII and IX[1]. The mainstay of treatment of haemophiliacs before 1974 was cryoprecipitate made from plasma obtained from UK volunteer blood donors, where each bag is made from one or two donations. This was supplemented by freeze dried intermediate NHS Factor VIII and Factor IX prepared from UK volunteer blood donors.

Table 1   Jaundice in haemophiliac patients in the United Kingdom

Year	Treated patients	No. of cases	Percent	
1969	1048	19	1.81	
1970	1041	25	2.40	
1971	1143	22	1.92	
1972	1191	17	1.42	
1973	1124	26	2.31	Commercial concentrates
1974	1634	85 (101)	5.20 (6.18)	first used
1975	1609	42 (51)	2.61 (3.17)	
1976	1886	56 (61)	2.97 (3.24)	Other commercial
1977	1968	50 (54)	2.54 (2.74)	concentrates
1978	2039	41 (47)	2.01 (2.30)	
1979	1935	33 (40)	1.70 (2.06)	

In response to the increased demand for Factor VIII, commercial freeze dried Factor VIII was imported from Europe and the USA to supplement NHS supplies. This was associated with an increase in the incidence of overt hepatitis from 2.31% in 1973 to 5.2% in 1974 (Table 1). Further studies showed in 1974-5 an attack rate of 17% in patients first treated with US commercial concentrate. Two types of hepatitis were observed; hepatitis B and what has since been shown to be non-A, non-B hepatitis with an incubation period of 6-70 days (mean 30.2 days)[2,3].

In 1976, three further brands of Factor VIII were licensed in the UK (Table 1). There are now six brands in use. Four brands manufactured in the USA from large pools of plasma (2-6000 litres) obtained by plasmapheresis of paid donors. These are high purity Factor VIII's made by modifications of the PEG/glycine buffer fractionation method[4]. A fifth brand is manufactured in Austria and is an intermediate type of Factor VIII. The sixth product is NHS intermediate concentrate prepared from plasma obtained from single donations of 200 ml each from UK volunteer donors. This means that the pool size of NHS Factor VIII may be larger (3500 donations per batch) than some batches of commercial factor where several litres of plasma is obtained by repeated plasmapheresis of one donor over a period of several weeks. This gives an advantage to commercial concentrate, and allows the use of large batches while keeping the number of donations per batch to a minimum. We do not know how this will affect the relative incidence of hepatitis associated with commercial Factor VIII compared with NHS concentrate, particularly as with whole blood transfusions there are 4 to 10 times the incidence of hepatitis associated with blood obtained from commercial, compared with voluntary donations[5].

TYPES OF HEPATITIS

Further observations have confirmed that two types of hepatitis are associated with transfusions of Factor VIII and IX. Table 2 summarises the data collected in the UK since 1974.

Hepatitis B

Despite the introduction of RIA screening of plasma donation for HB_sAg in 1975, a significant amount of both symptomatic and symptomless hepatitis B still occurs associated with commercial and NHS Factor VIII transfusions[6].

Table 2   Hepatitis B and non-B hepatitis related to factor VIII
transfusions in the UK

Year	Batches	Non-B hepatitis	Hepatitis B (overt)	Total hepatitis	Total transfused	Product
1974-5	Q-V (6)	45 (14.6%)	26 (8.4%)	62	308F*	Commercial
1975	W-Z4(7)	10 (7.4%)	2 (1.5%)	12	136F	Commercial
1975-6	K1-K12	13 (10.9%)	4 (3.4%)	17	119F	Commercial
1977	NS	33 (1.68)	17 (0.56)	50 (2.54)	1968A**	All
1978	NS	34 (1.66)	8 (0.39)	47 (2.01)	2039A	All
1979	NS	29 (1.49)	4 (0.20)	33 (1.7)	1935A	All
TOTAL		164	61			

*F - first transfused

**A - all transfused

Table 3   Prevalence of hepatitis B antibody Anti-HB$_s$ and Anti-HB$_c$
in Oxford haemophiliacs

Treatment group	Product transfused	Anti-HB$_c$ or Anti-HB$_s$ positive±	Anti-HB$_c$ and Anti-HB$_s$ negative	HB$_s$Ag carriers	Total
Haemophilia 'A' Severe*	NHS + commercial VIII concentrate	112 (86%)	8 (6.0%)	3 (2.3%)	130 #
Haemophilia 'A' Mild*	Blood or cryoprecipitate	0	17	0	17
Christmas disease	NHS IX concentrate	15 (88%)	0	0	16 <>

* Severity of coagulation defect

7/130 patients with doubtful antibody status had antibody passively
acquired from transfused concentrate

± 'Ausab' RIA Positive ratio > 20

  Negative ratio < 3.0

  Doubtful ratio < 20 and > 3.0

  Anti-HB$_c$ 'Corab' RIA

<> 1/16 patients with doubtful antibody status

Table 3 shows the results of a survey carried out at the Oxford Haemophilia Centre of the prevalence of hepatitis B surface (anti-HB$_s$) and core (anti-HB$_c$) antibodies in different groups of patients by radio-immunoassay (RIA). A positive result is obtained from the ratio:

counts per minute in the test serum
counts per minute in the negative control serum

A positive result was taken to be a ratio of > 20. Values below this may be due to passively acquired antibody from transfusions of factor VIII or IX (< 20 > 3.0). Ratio < 3.0 were considered to be negative (AUSAB RIA test - Abbott Laboratories Ltd.).

The results indicate that -

1) 75-80% of patients with severe Factor VIII or IX deficiency are anti-HB$_s$ positive, and are therefore immune to reinfection.

2) The proportion of carriers of hepatitis B virus (HBV) (3/130 or 2.3%) is no higher than in non-haemophiliacs with a similar exposure to HBV. Therefore, chronic hepatitis associated with HBV infection is not a major cause of chronic liver disease in British haemophiliacs.

3) Infection with HBV is highly correlated with the use of large pool concentrate, both NHS and commercial. Most of these patients started treatment before RIA testing of donations for fractionation of plasma was introduced in 1975. Prospective studies of patients at Oxford after first transfusion of concentrate suggest that the attack rate for hepatitis B may have declined markedly, e.g. two out of eight patients (25%) showed serological evidence of symptomless hepatitis B infection after transfusions of up to 5000 Factor VIII units. Prior to 1975 the rate was probably 80-90%[3].

4) Many haemophiliacs with severe coagulation defect are exposed to hepatitis B infection before the age of 10 years. A high proportion of infection in young children is symptomless, as few give a history of symptomatic illness compatible with hepatitis B.

5)   Patients with mild coagulation defects (VIII > 2%) often do not require regular Factor VIII therapy and only require concentrate to cover an operation or other major accident. Thus they do not receive treatment with concentrate until they are 30-40 years old when undergoing an operation or other procedure. They are then more likely to suffer from symtomatic hepatitis B than if they had contracted it as a child.

Non-A, Non-B Hepatitis

The acute illness is clinically mild with an incubation period of 6-70 days and is clinically indistinguishable from hepatitis A and B. Of a total of 138 cases where transfusion history was known, 103 have been associated with first transfusion of Factor VIII or IX concentrate[6]. Only seven cases have been associated with transfusions of cryoprecipitate. Each patient had received cryoprecipitate from between 50 and 100 plasma donations in the 6 months prior to the onset of actue hepatitis. This suggests a low contamination ratio for cryoprecipitate made from UK volunteer donors for non-A, non-B hepatitis. Secondary symptomatic cases have not been reported in household contacts in contrast to hepatitis B, where six secondary cases have occurred since 1974.

We have recently published evidence[7], based on the occurrence of multiple attacks of hepatitis in haemophiliacs, in favour of the existence of at least two types of non-A, non-B hepatitis associated with transfusions of Factor VIII. One type is associated with US sourced commercial products. The second is associated with NHS Factor VIII and European commercial products. This association of different serotypes with different brands of Factor VIII is probably related to the different fractionation process used in the preparation of US commercial Factor VIII compared with NHS Factor VIII and European. The US products are made from modifications of the PEG/glycine fractionation method[4].

The early reported cases associated with US commercial concentrates had a high attack rate (14.6%). These were patients receiving their first transfusion of concentrate. However, the current cumulative attack rate is almost 1.7% of the total patients treated in 1979 in the UK (Table 2). Studies of patients receiving first transfusions of concentrate suggest that the attack rate for non-A, non-B hepatitis has remained unchanged since 1974[6]. This is in marked contrast to the risk of contracting hepatitis B which has fallen since the introduction of RIA screening of plasma donations for HB_sAg.

Symptomless Non-A, Non-B Hepatitis

It was shown in a recent publication[7] that a patient was 20 times more likely to contract symptomatic non-A, non-B hepatitis with the first batch of concentrate he received than after a second or subsequent batch[7]. This suggested that symptomless patients were protected from contracting hepatitis after transfusion of second or subsequent batches of concentrate due to the acquisition of immunity from a symptomless infection associated with the first batch of concentrate transfused. Recent evidence suggests that the overall attack rate including symptomless infection is about 80–90% with the first batch of concentrate received[6,8].

Table 4. Factor VIII associated hepatitis: commercial and NHS brands. Attack rates in patients receiving one product in a treatment year.

Year	Brand	Cases of hepatitis Non-B (overt)	Overt B	Total overt hepatitis	Total transfused	Ratio Comm/NHS Non-B	B
1977	*Comm	3 (2.67)	2 (1.78)	5 (4.46)	112)		
					)	4.76	0.79
	*NHS	1 (0.56)	4 (2.23)	5 (2.79)	179)		
1978	Comm	14 (7.7)	1 (0.5)	15 (8.3)	180)		
					)	19.7	0.79
	NHS	1 (0.39)	2 (0.63)	3 (0.96)	313)		
1979	Comm	10 (6.30)	1 (0.63)	11 (6.96)	158)		
					)	21.73	*n/s
	NHS	1 (0.29)	0	1 (0.29)	342)		

* Comm   –   Commercial concentrate
* NHS   –   National Health Service (Intermediate) factor VIII concentrate
* n/s   –   not significant
Figures in brackets equal percentages

The attack rates for symptomatic hepatitis for patients treated with one brand of concentrate in any year suggest that there is an increased risk from commercial Factor VIII compared with NHS Factor VIII (see Table 4), but no firm conclusion can be drawn until prospective studies have been carried out.

Complications

Most cases of non-A, non-B hepatitis are mild illnesses. Six cases have been reported as 'severe'. Two patients have died in the acute stage of the disease, but there were complicating factors in both instances.

Acute Fulminating Hepatitis

This has not been reported in our survey, but occured after transfusions of Factor IX to non-haemophiliac patients with chronic liver disease not associated with viral hepatitis[9,10]. The Factor IX was used to achieve normal clotting factor levels prior to liver biopsy or other operative procedure. In one episode[9], three out of four patients who contracted non-A, non-B hepatitis died of acute fulminating hepatitis. The use of Factor IX concentrate is, therefore, strongly contraindicated in non-haemophiliac patients until a means is found of rendering these products safe from the risk of acute hepatitis.

Chronic Liver Disease

About 25-40% of haemophiliacs on regular Factor VIII therapy have persistently elevated serum aminotransferase levels for periods of at least one year[11,12]. Most of these patients are symptomless. However, a few have clinical features suggestive of chronic liver disease, but the ethical problems associated with the indications for liver biopsy have meant that few patients have so far undergone this procedure. About 40 patients have undergone biopsy in the UK and approximately 50% of these have histological evidence of chronic persistent hepatitis[13,14]. Other patients showed evidence of chronic liver disease or cirrhosis. The histological changes showed no correlation with the degree of disturbance of the serum enzyme levels. The only common factor was regular treatment with Factor VIII concentrate. Most of the patients in this group are children or young adults, though the age range at Oxford is 6-70 years. It seems likely that some patients will develop severe chronic liver disease over the next 10 years. Further data relating to problems will be given in later papers in this Symposium. There is no evidence that household contacts of haemophiliacs are liable to develop chronic liver disease.

Since less than 5% of British haemophiliacs are carriers of HBV, it is likely that most of the chronic hepatitis is a sequel to infection with non-A, non-B hepatitis virus(es). A carrier state similar to that for hepatitis B has been recently shown to exist for at least 6 years[15]. There is as yet no evidence that any other factor is involved, such as hypersensitivity to components in the transfused concentrate or constant re-exposure to toxic chemicals in the concentrate. One patient suffered from five successive attacks of acute hepatitis following five successive transfusion episodes several months apart[16]. Each episode was followed by the liver function tests returning to normal. The last episode was partially alleviated by treatment with steroids. The authors suggested that the patient concerned suffered from hypersensitivity to a component in the transfused concentrate. These features are in marked contrast to those associated with viral hepatitis.

There is, therefore, a high risk from the use of Factor VIII or IX concentrate that the patient will contract non-A, non-B hepatitis, and a 20-30% chance of resultant chronic hepatitis, together with a smaller risk of hepatitis B. Most severe haemophiliacs in the UK have now been exposed to these viruses. Until tests are available for these agents, the possibility of using small pool concentrate or a wider use of cryoprecipitate should be considered for patients with mild coagulation defects requiring treatment to cover surgery or other major treatment. These patients are infrequently treated and run a high risk of transfusion hepatitis if concentrate is used for the first time.

REFERENCES

1. Biggs, R. (1974). Jaundice and antibodies against factors VIII and IX in patients treated for haemophilia and Christmas disease in the United Kingdom. Br. J. Haematol., 26, 313

2. Craske, J., Dilling, N. and Stern, D. (1975). An outbreak of hepatitis associated with intravenous infection of factor VIII concentrate. Lancet, ii, 221

3. Craske, J., Kirk, P., Cohen, B. and Vandervelde, Elise, M., (1978). Commercial factor VIII associated hepatitis, 1974-5, in the United Kingdom: A retrospective survey. J. Hyg. Camb., 80, 327

4. Brinkhous, K.M., Shanbrom, E., Roberts, H.R., Webster, W.P., Fekete, L. and Wagner, R.H. (1968). A new high potency glycine-precipitated anti-haemophilic factor (AHF) concentrate: Treatment of classical haemophilia and haemophilia with inhibitors. J. Am. Med. Assoc., 205, 613

5. Goldfield, M., Black, H.C., Bill, J., Srihongse, S., and Pizzuti, W. (1975). The consequences of administering blood pre-tested for HB$_s$Ag. by third generation techniques: A progress report. Am. J. Med. Sci., 270, 335

6. U.K. Haemophilia Hepatitis Working Party (1977-9). Unpublished observation.

7. Craske, J., Spooner, R.J.D. and Vandervelde, Elise, M. (1978). Evidence in favour of the existence of at least two types of factor VIII associated non-B hepatitis. Lancet, ii, 1051

8. Sugg, U., Schmidt, M. and Schneider, W. (1980). Clotting factors and non-A, non-B hepatitis. N. Engl. J. Med., 303, 943

9. Wyke, R.J., Tsique, K.N., Thornton, A., White, Y., Portman, B., Das, P.K., Zuckerman, A.J. and Williams, R. (1979). Transmission of non-A, non-B hepatitis to chimpanzees by factor IX concentrates after fatal complications in patients with chronic liver disease. Lancet, i, 520

10. Delarge, C. and Legrace, R. (1974). Hepatite associée à la prise de Konyne: Observation clinico-pathologique de 10 cas. Med. Canada. 103, 1207

11. Mannuci, P.M., Capitano, A., del Ninno, E., Colombo, M., Paneti, F., and Ruggeri, Z.M. (1975). Asymptomatic liver disease in haemophiliacs. J. Clin. Pathol., 28, 620

12. U.K. Haemophilia Hepatitis Working Party (1979). Unpublished observation.

13. Lesesne, H.R., Morgan, J.E., Blatt, P.M., Webster, W.P., and

Roberts, H.R. (1977). Liver biopsy in haemophilia. Ann. Intern. Med., 86, 703

14. Preston, F.E., Triger, D.R., Underwood, J.C.E., Bardhan, A., Mitchell, V.E., Stewart, R.M. and Blackburn, E.K. (1978). Percutaneous liver biopsy and chronic liver disease in haemophiliacs. Lancet, ii, 592

15. Tabor, E., Seeff, L.B. and Gerety, R.J. (1980). Chronic non-A, non-B hepatitis carrier state. Transmissable agent documented in one patient over a six-year period. N. Engl., J. Med., 303, 140

16. Myers, T.J., Tembrevilla-Zubiri, C.L., Klatsky, A.U. and Rickles, F.R. (1980). Recurrent acute hepatitis following the use of factor VIII concentrates. Blood, 55, 748

Discussion

Prof. MacSween: I was not quite sure about the difference in incidence of hepatitis between the commercial concentrates and the NHS concentrates.

Dr. Craske: The problem is that it looks as if there is a much higher incidence in overt cases, but the difficulty is that in the total population we have studied there are so many patients who have had treatment before. That is why I was a bit guarded about the interpretation.

Prof. MacSween: This would provide evidence, as you suggest, that there might be a number of different agents responsible for causing the hepatitis, and it might be explicable on that basis. Have you seen any patients who have been treated with the NHS concentrate and then subsequently had the commerical and then developed overt hepatitis?

Dr. Craske: Yes. This was actually reported 2 years ago in the Lancet. We have a group of about 20 patients who had multiple attacks and the evidence may be interpreted as suggesting that these patients experienced 2 attacks of non-A, non-B hepatitis, and that they could have experienced 3 agents at least. Interestingly enough the incubation periods seemed to all be of this short type. One other thing, which has been reported recently, has been a case where a patient had 5 episodes of jaundice after successive transfusions of concentrate, in which this was thought to be related to allergy to some product in the Factor VIII. The interesting feature of this was that the incubation period in successive exposures got less and less until at the final exposure the incubation period was about 3 days. In each case the liver function test, returned to normal after a month or two, so that this would seem to be a different type of hepatitis to the one we have been describing today. When the report came up I looked at the incubation periods in our multiple cases and the second episode of hepatitis did not, in most cases, have a shorter incubation period than the first. Thus I do not think our repeated cases can be explained on allergy.

Prof. MacSween: I suppose the other possibility is that in non-A, non-B hepatitis where there are fluctuations in liver function tests there may just be a coincidental change in transaminase levels.

Dr. Craske: That is true, but these cases all had overt jaundice. These were mostly mildly affected patients, and in a quarter of the cases liver function tests had returned to normal. We do not seem to see this very often with severely affected ones. This may just be that they get very heavy exposure, and therefore they perhaps get infections very close together. We also looked at the incidence of hepatitis-A antibody in haemophiliacs at Oxford and there is no correlation with exposure to concentrates at all. The incidence of antibodies is exactly what we would expect from a comparable group of non-haemophiliacs in Oxford who experienced hepatitis-A infection by other routes.

We have two reports of hepatitis-A in haemophilia-B patients at Oxford where it seems just remotely possible that they could have acquired it from concentrate. We are looking into this possibility because we do seem to have a cluster. But whether this is related to the concentrate remains to be seen but it is theoretically possible.

Prof. Stewart: As I understand it, non-A, non-B causes chronic hepatitis. They keep on getting it and they keep on with their abnormalities in the liver function tests. How can this be squared with the explanation regarding the severely affected patients that have been exposed and have become infected?

Dr. Craske: The point is that being an infective disease, it needs one exposure to get infected. After exposure to this infection the patient presumably gets a chronic inflammatory process in the liver, which is why he gets persistence, as evidenced by the abnormal liver function tests. In addition there is better evidence which will be demonstrated by the people who will describe the abnormalities of the liver biopsy.

Prof. Stewart: How can this be squared with the severe cases who do not seem to have it?

Dr. Craske: They do not get a fresh attack of jaundice. That is what I meant. We do not see fresh cases of overt non-A, non-B hepatitis in patients who have been transfused with so much concentrate that they have experienced all the possible infective agents present in this material.

Prof. Stewart: Have they still got abnormal liver funtion?

Dr. Craske: A high proportion of them have. Some of them will get better within 6 months and some a year. One of the problems is the length of time which is the normal lifespan of this infection? We do not know, and it seems to be a bit longer than other types of hepatitis.

Prof. MacSween: The difficulty is that one may be dealing with a patient who has a background of chronic liver disease, and whether another attack of hepatitis or jaundice in that patient should be equated with a reinfection or an exacerbation of acute -on- chronic episodes presents a lot of problems.

Dr. Craske: There is a small amount of cases, which I have not described, where we get jaundice in patients who are considered to have chronic liver disease, and we do not know what it is due to; there are many possible causes. I have deliberately excluded these. It was only in two cases where the epidemiological evidence suggested that it was related to the transfusion episode and where the director concerned was convinced that the clinical symptoms would fit this syndrome. The confirmation of this is the constant number of incidents we get and the constant situation where it occurs.

2 Viruses causing hepatitis

C. H. Cameron

The infectious agents to be considered here are the human hepatitis viruses. Although there are other viruses which may sometimes involve the liver, these do not represent a practical problem in the present context, and will not be mentioned further.

The hepatitis viruses include the well-known hepatitis A and hepatitis B viruses together with at least one agent, probably more, causing what is at present know as "non-A, non-B" hepatitis.

In hepatitis A the maximum faecal excretion of virus occurs some days before the onset of illness. Antibody to the virus appears and may be detected in the blood later in the clinical illness and in convalescence. A transient viraemia is probably usual, but there is no simple screening test for potentially infectious blood donations. Fortunately however post-transfusion hepatitis A, although a theoretical risk, is quite rare in this country and I do not know of any proven case of hepatitis A attributable to the use of factor VIII preparations.

The diagnosis of non-A, non-B hepatitis requires by definition the exclusion of the diagnosis of hepatitis A or hepatitis B, but beyond this we can dismiss hepatitis A as unimportant in the context of therapy in haemophilia.

The hepatitis B virus (HBV), which is of considerable importance in blood transfusion and the use of blood products, is fortunately better endowed with markers of infectivity which can be demonstrated in blood samples by laboratory tests. The HBV particle, which is about 42 nm in diameter, carries on its surface the most important antigen from the point of view of practical screening of donations. This so-called 'surface-antigen' (HB_sAg) actually possesses several antigenic determinants which include amongst others the common 'a' antigen and either the 'd' or the 'y' subtype-specific antigens. The reason why we are able to detect the great majority of infectious blood donations, even those containing very small amounts of infectious virus, is that HB_sAg also occurs in the form of 22 nm particles which vastly outnumber the complete infectious virus particles. Without this huge excess of small particles we would have difficulty in detecting even the most highly infectious bloods by testing for the presence of HB_sAg. Virus isolation in tissue culture, which for many viruses is the most sensitive method of detection, is not a practical possibility in the case of the hepatitis viruses. This unusually large amount of circulating virus antigen, which is sometimes found at concentrations as high as 0.5 mg/ml, is present at detectable levels almost throughout the period when the blood is infectious (except for a short time during the incubation period, and sometimes also in convalescence) and is the most valuable marker of infectivity, and all blood donations in this country and many others are screened for the presence of HBs antigen. The more sensitive the test used for HB_sAg detection, the more nearly one approaches the ideal of eliminating all infectious donations. There is however no reason to suppose that radioimmunoassay methods would detect all the dangerous blood donations missed by the less sensitive methods; it is necessary to bind several million ^{125}I-labelled antibody molecules in order to give a significant count rate as measured in a counting time of a few minutes.

Antibody to surface antigen (anti-HBs) develops in most persons recovering from hepatitis B, although this is very variable in amount and in its time of appearance after infection - sometimes as much as a year.

The inner core of the virus carries a different antigenic determinant on its protein shell, the 'core antigen' (HB_cAg), and antibody to this antigen (anti-HBc) develops much more predictably, and to a higher titre, appearing towards the end of the incubation period when surface antigen is becoming detectable.

A further antigen, the 'e' antigen (HB_eAg), is associated with the presence of infectious virus particles, although it appears to occur largely as a 'free' or 'soluble' protein antigen. It has a strong association with the degree of infectivity of the blood, and its disappearance, and the appearance of anti-HB_e antibody is associated with a reduction in circulating infectious virus particles irrespective of the total HB_sAg content.

Chronic carriers of hepatitis B virus occur, and represent a very important reservior of infection. Broadly speaking they fall into three groups. Those positive for HB_eAg have highly infectious blood, and represent some risk to their close contacts. Those positive for anti-HB_e have less infectious blood, and do not readily transmit the infection to their close contacts. In some carriers neither HB_eAg nor anti-HB_e are detectable, and these appear to be in an intermediate phase. However, even the blood of anti-HB_e positive carriers is by no means safe when transfused by the pint.

In the case of 'non-A, non-B hepatitis' our knowledge is at the moment much more rudimentary and incomplete. Most of our present information is of an epidemiological nature, as outlined by Dr. Craske, although experimental work in chimpanzees has contributed valuable additional data.

It seems quite likely that there are at least two agents causing non-A, non-B hepatitis, and that one has a relatively long, and one a relatively short incubation period. Although there may also be dose-related variations in incubation period with a single infectious agent, there is some confirmatory evidence for the existence of more than one agent derived from cross-challenge experiments in chimpanzees.

Attention is being directed in several laboratories to the possibility that there might be markers of infectivity in the blood for these non-A, non-B agents, as in the case of hepatitis B. If this were so then it might be possible to detect the blood donations likely to transmit these agents. There is no reason to expect that such markers should necessarily be present, (hepatitis B is after all rather unusual amongst viruses), nor have we any reason to expect that they would be present in amounts sufficent to allow detection of the majority of dangerous donations by means of mass screening procedures. However if this does prove to be the case then we shall fortunately be in the position to reduce the incidence of non-A, non-B hepatitis following blood transfusion or Factor VIII administration. There have been a few preliminary encouraging reports from workers in various countries, using immunodiffusion and related techniques, but it must be said that this work is still in its infancy and is as yet lacking in confirmation on a wide scale. We shall have to wait and see what emerges as the work proceeds.

The subject of chronic infection and liver damage due to non-A, non-B agents will be discussed by others presently.

Returning now to hepatitis B, and the laboratory testing of plasma pools and Factor VIII concentrates, some of our past experiences may be of interest. In 1974 three batches of Factor VIII, having passed the manufacturers' tests, were imported from the USA. In those days it was common practice to screen the individual contributors to the plasma pools for the presence of HB_sAg by the counter immunoelectrophoretic (CIEP) method, and to test the final product by radioimmunoassay (RIA). The pool sizes were such that, as a result of dilution (ignoring the effects of antibody-positive packs in the pool), the RIA testing of the final product was only likely to be positive if a pack was included in the pool which should have been detected by the initial (CIEP) screening. The RIA, although a much more sensitive test, was in effect only a check on the original screening after the large dilution involved in the pooling. The RIA most widely used at the time was the commercial product Ausria 1, which was not a particularly sensitive RIA by modern standards. The three batches of factor VIII were also tested in the UK by the National Institute for Biological Standards and Control, as is customary. One of the batches gave a borderline result; in one test run it gave counts just above the 'cut-off', and in another test run, just below. We were sent samples of the three batches, and tested them in our own RIA system, which was of higher sensitivity than Ausria 1. The results are shown superimposed on titration of an HB_sAg positive serum of high titre (Figure 1), and the non-specific binding given with normal human serum is indicated.

Of the three samples tested (A, B and C), the suspect, C, gave a strong positive reaction corresponding to an HB_sAg concentration of about 15 ng/ml, thus coinciding with the limit of sensitivity of the Ausria 1 test. Samples A and B were also positive, but at the lower levels of about 1.5 ng/ml and 0.35 ng/ml respectively.

It was reasonable that clinicians dealing with cases of haemophilia should have access to this material as long as the risk of hepatitis B infection was known; the risk of infection could be balanced against the risks involved in witholding this material in a severe bleeding crisis. However, in order to provide a safer product, it was decided that from September 1975 onwards all donations should be tested individually by RIA before pooling for Factor VIII production.

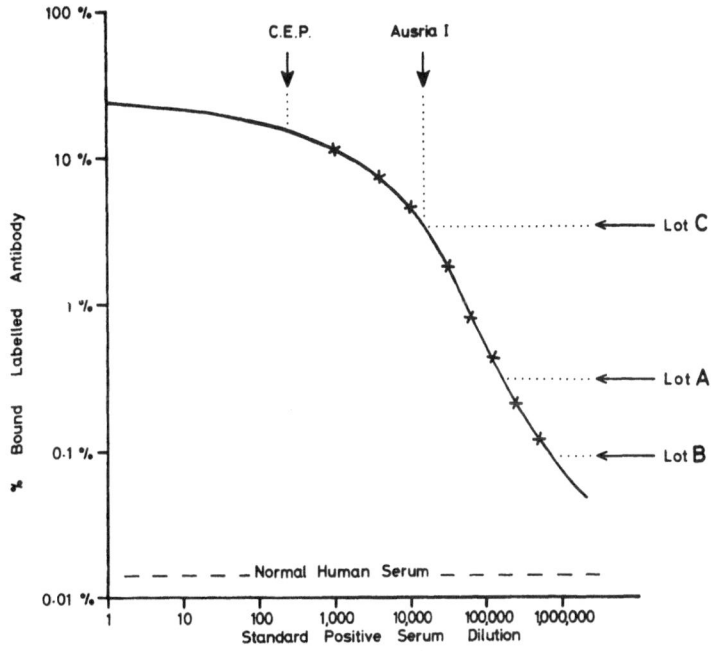

Figure 1   Titration curve showing the binding of radiolabelled antibody
with a series of dilutions of an HBsAg positive serum. The
binding given by samples A, B and C is indicated together
with the end-points of the other detection methods

In order to increase the sensitivity of our HB_sAg testing of blood
products, we used a modification of the method of Harris, Semar and
Johnson[1], in which HB_sAg was concentrated by PEG precipitation after
preliminary digestion of the other proteins with pepsin. We used an
additional high pH trypsin digestion stage after the low pH pepsin digestion
stage in order to so cleave any anti-HB_s antibody bound to the antigen that
the antigenic binding sites would be unmasked and the HB_sAg would be
more readily detected in the subsequent RIA test. This enzymatic digestion
and PEG precipitation procedure followed by RIA (EDPP-RIA) was used in
testing a number of factor VIII concentrates and immunoglobulin
preparations. The results of these tests are included in the data (Table 1)
relating the incidence of hepatitis B and non-B in recipients, to the batches
of Factor VIII received. A lower incidence of hepatitis B is associated with
the batches in which the individual donations were screened by RIA before
pooling.

Table 1   Incidence of overt hepatitis in recipients of Factor VIII prepared from CIEP or RIA screened donations.

Screening method	No. of batches	Positive EDPP-RIA	Patients exposed	Non-B Hep cases (%)	Hep B cases (%)
CIEP	2	Not tested	91	9 (9.9)	10 (11.0)
CIEP	4	4	213	36 (16.9)	15 (7.0)
RIA	7	0	136	10 (7.4)	2 (1.5)

Laboratory testing for the safety of the factor VIII concentrates inevitably has its limitations.   As with other products, such as killed vaccines or immunoglobulin preparations, the ultimate test of infectivity is the administration of the material to large numbers of human subjects.

REFERENCE

1.   Harris, R.B., Semar, M. and Johnson, A.J. (1977). Detection of hepatitis B surface antigen in potentially contaminated human plasma and plasma fractions. J. Lab. Clin. Med., 90, 1107

Discussion

Prof. Stewart: Are you assuming that the only source of hepatitis-B infection is transfusion material?

Dr. Cameron: No.   The change in the figures is probably largely due to the more careful regulation of the raw materials from which Factor VIII is prepared.   There may be other variables in the system, but I can see no reason to doubt that we have produced a reduction in hepatitis-B infections from Factor VIII preparations, both in the UK and elsewhere.

Anonymous: Have you any advice to offer on accepting as potential blood donors those who have already had hepatitis-A?

Dr. Cameron: I think that the clinical policy now is to accept people with a history of jaundice in the distant past, provided that they pass all the standard tests for surface antigens, and to exclude people with a recent history of jaundice until such time as they have been shown to be clear of antigen, and I think in the case of recent jaundice not to reinstate them on to the panel until they have shown evidence of producing antibodies to surface antigen. As far as hepatitis-A is concerned, I do not think that there is anything in the regulations specifically connected with hepatitis-A, just the regulations concerned with the history of unspecified jaundice - that I mentioned. As far as I know hepatitis-A does not represent any form of long-term risk in that a person who suffers from hepatitis-A, there is virtually no evidence that they might become a chronic carrier of hepatitis-A, and remain infectious for years to come.

3

Clinical, immunological and histological aspects of non-A, non-B hepatitis in haemophiliacs

H. C. Thomas, M. Bamber and P. B. A. Kernoff

Although the incidence of symptomatic hepatitis associated with jaundice in patients with congenital coagulation disorders is low[1,2], several reports have demonstrated that many of these patients have asymptomatic liver disease. Mannucci et al., in 1975[3] showed increased transaminases in more than 40% of haemophiliacs and Levine et al., in 1976[4] found similar abnormalities in 68% of patients. The latter study included 33 intensively treated patients from the Royal Free Hospital who had received cryoprecipitate only and who had a 48.5% prevalence of abnormal liver function tests. More recently, in a survey of 76 patients with severe haemophilia A (Factor VIII < 1%) registered at the Royal Free Hospital Haemophilia Centre, 92% were found to have abnormal aspartate transaminase levels on random testing[5]. The prevalence of abnormalities was similar in patients who had received NHS concentrate only (100%) and those who had received commercial Factor VIII preparations (96%), but slightly lower in those who had received cryoprecipitate only (80%). Seven untreated patients with mild haemophilia had normal liver function tests. Although the number of patients who had received NHS concentrate or cryoprecipitate only was smaller than the number who had received commercial concentrate, and patients receiving cryoprecipitate only were in general transfused less frequently than those receiving concentrate. This evidence suggests that infusion of large donor pool Factor VIII concentrates, whether of NHS or commercial origin, is a major cause of liver function test abnormalities. This conclusion is supported by the finding of a higher prevalence of abnormal tests now than in 1976, when a larger proportion of our patients was maintained exclusively on cryoprecipitate.

It seems probable that transfusion-transmitted viral hepatitis is responsible for liver function test abnormalities in the majority of patients. For several reasons, it is unlikely that hepatitis B virus (HBV) is the main causative agent. HBV infection is not commonly followed by sustained abnormalities of liver function tests and, when it is, HB_s antigen is usually detectable in the blood. Some patients have intrahepatic HBV infection without detectable HB_s antigen[6,7] but these patients usually have detectable antibody to the core of the virus (anti-HB_c) without antibody to the surface coat protein (anti-HB_s). Haemophiliacs only rarely exhibit these patterns of serological abnormalities, and only occasionally develop acute HBV infection. The low incidence of the latter is probably in part related to the introduction of sensitive radioimmunoassays for HB_s antigen in the screening of blood donors, which has considerably reduced the incidence of HBV infection. It is also relevant, however, that a majority of haemophiliacs have detectable anti-HB_s in their blood[5,8]. Whether this represents active immunisation following previous sub-clinical infection or merely passive immunisation by globulin contained in transfused blood products is unknown. In either event, the presence of anti-HB_s in the blood could confer protection to infection with HBV.

With the development of serological techniques for the identification of type A and B hepatitis viruses, it has become evident that additional hepatitis viruses exist. These have been provisionally designated the non-A, non-B (NANB) hepatitis viruses and appear to be responsible for approximately 90% of post-transfusion hepatitis[9,10,11]. It seems probable that NANB viruses are responsible for the majority of liver function test abnormalities seen in haemophiliacs. There is evidence of more than one type of NANB virus. In one study a drug addict was reported as suffering from four separate attacks of hepatitis – one type A, one type B and, in addition, two further episodes[12]. Additional evidence also stems from experiments performed in chimpanzees. Animals given Factor IX concentrates developed NANB hepatitis with an incubation period of 10 weeks. These animals were then given Factor VIII concentrate and, 10-14 days after infusion, developed a second episode of NANB hepatitis[13]. Morphological studies of the liver during these episodes of short and long incubation NANB hepatitis suggested cytologically distinct patterns[14,15]. There may be other causes for the elevation of transaminases following Factor VIII infusion. One group of authors have suggested that episodes of hepatitis in some haemophilic patients may represent allergic phenomena secondary to a protein contaminant of Factor VIII concentrate[16].

FEATURES OF POST-TRANSFUSION HEPATITIS IN HAEMOPHILIACS

To more fully document the natural history of liver function test changes following exposure to Factor VIII concentrates, detailed studies were carried out in nine patients with haemophilia and one with von Willebrand's disease who developed acute post-transfusion hepatitis. The patients were followed for periods ranging from 6 to 30 months. All the patients had normal pre-transfusion liver function tests, and seven were receiving concentrates for the first time[17]. In the six patients who received a single infusion in the 3 months prior to the development of hepatitis, the incubation period was found to be between 1 and 4 weeks. In the remaining four patients the infusate responsible for transmission of the infection could not be established with certainty although the interval between the last infusion and the onset of elevated transaminase was also 1-4 weeks. This incubation period is shorter than that described in non-haemophilic patients developing NANB hepatitis after blood transfusion, but is in accord with other reports of non-B hepatitis in haemophiliacs[18,19]. In general, non-haemophilic patients exhibit mean incubation periods of 6-8 weeks[20,21].

Seven patients were symptomatic. Symptoms included lethargy, nausea, general malaise, abdominal discomfort and jaundice; and generally lasted a few weeks only. In some patients, symptoms recurred after initially subsiding, particularly at the time of rises of transaminase. In one patient, the symptoms were severe and persistent and eventually, 7 months after the onset of the illness, necessitated steroid therapy. Four patients exhibited a mild degree of splenomegaly but there was no significant enlargement of the liver. None of the patients had radiographic or ultrasonographic evidence of portal hypertension or oesophageal varices.

The biochemical picture was characteristic. Aspartate transaminase (AST) rose rapidly to a peak value and then fluctuated rapidly with a periodicity of 14-20 days (Figure 1).

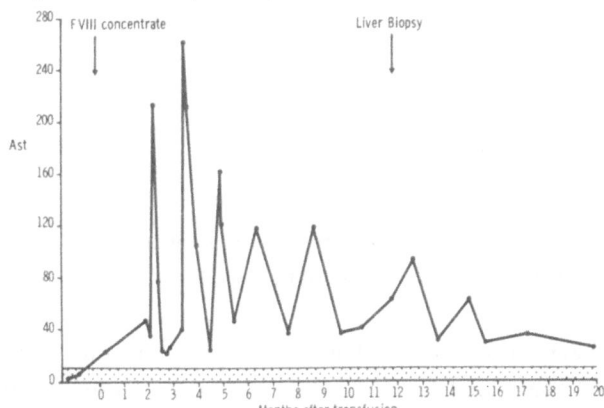

Figure 1

In some cases the AST would fall to normal values for 1-2 days and then rise rapidly to moderately elevated levels. In others, the fluctuating pattern was superimposed on a mild persistent elevation. The pattern of AST abnormality was similar in patients receiving different quantities of factor VIII. The peak elevation was usually within the first month and ranged from 75 to 1100 IU/l (normal less than 15 IU/l). Six of our patients still had elevated transaminase levels 6 months after the onset of the illness. At this time, bilirubin and alkaline phosphatase concentrations were normal.

Five patients underwent liver biopsy - three during the acute phase of their illness (during the first 6 months) and two during the chronic phase (after 6 months). The former were performed because the aetiology of the liver function test abnormalities was not entirely clear. The biopsies taken during the acute phase showed the typical features of actue hepatitis. Of the two biopsies taken during the chronic phase of the illness, one showed chronic persistent and one chronic active hepatitis. The most prominent histological feature was a severe mononuclear cell infiltration of the hepatic lobule without marked liver cell necrosis (Figure 2).

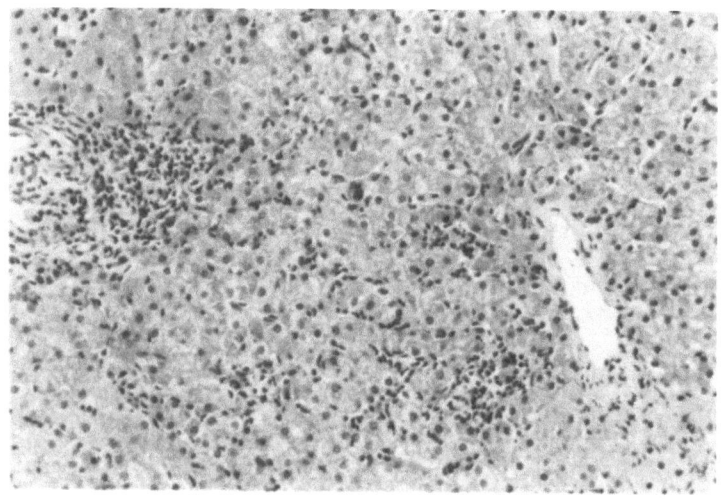

Figure 2   Chronic active hepatitis with prominent mononuclear cell
                infiltration of the hepatic lobules

This picture was similar to Epstein-Barr virus infection. Bile duct damage similar to that described by Poulsen and Christoffersen (1978)[22] was noted but not thought to be particularly prominent or specific for NANB hepatitis.

None of the patients showed serological evidence of acute infection with hepatitis A or B, Epstein-Barr or cytomegalovirus. None of the patients with chronic hepatitis (abnormal AST for greater than 6 months) had abnormalities of immunoglobulin concentrations or autoantibodies. The majority of patients had evidence of circulating immune complexes detectable by the C1q binding assay. This confirms an earlier report by McVerry et. al.[23] (1977) in which 94% of a group of haemophiliacs attending this centre were found to have circulating immune complexes, 55% of these patients having abnormal AST. In our study the level of C1q binding activity and the degree of complement activation was not significantly greater than that found in patients with other types of acute and chronic hepatitis[24]. The accumulation of large immune complexes in patients with acute and chronic liver disease is probably a reflection of impairment of the hepatic component of the reticuloendothelial system rather than a specific feature of the disease[25].

Three groups of workers have published data describing an immunoprecipitin test for NANB hepatitis[26-28]. These serological systems have generally been described in post-transfusion hepatitis exhibiting incubation periods between 6 and 13 weeks. The sera from our patients were examined by immunodiffusion for antigen/antibody systems, testing early-phase sera against serially-obtained 'convalescent phase' sera. Six patients demonstrated NANB associated antigen – three of these patients subsequently developed antibody. A further patient demonstrated antibody without preceding demonstrable antigenaemia. Antigenaemia was usually brief, being in most cases present in a single sample. The development of antibody did not signify recovery as regards normalisation of liver function tests. The relationship of this antigen/antibody system to NANB hepatitis is under continuing investigation to determine the specificity of the association.

SUMMARY

The data from our prospective study suggests that patients receiving Factor VIII concentrates (commercial and NHS) for the first time run a high risk of developing acute NANB hepatitis. The incidence of chronicity in our study was higher than that observed by others. Six of our patients had persistently elevated transaminases at 6 months, whereas in previous studies (usually of non-haemophiliac patients) chronicity rates of between 25-50%[9,29-31] have been found. The high attack rate with a high incidence of chronicity suggests that the majority of the haemophiliac population exposed to Factor VIII concentrates will develop chronic hepatitis, at least as regards the definition of transaminase abnormalities persisting for longer than 6 months.

In a larger series of biopsies in this patient group we found 5 of 12 patients (42%) biopsied during the chronic phase to have chronic active hepatitis. Although the prognosis of this lesion following NANB hepatitis is unknown, it should be noted that a similar lesion associated with chronic hepatitis B virus infection is progressive and, in a proportion of patients, ultimately results in the development of cirrhosis and its attendant complications. Most of our patients had liver biopsies carried out within 6-36 months of the recognised onset of transaminase abnormality. Only one patient was found to have evidence of cirrhosis, which indicates a relatively slow rate of progression. The potentially serious nature of the disease, however, make close clinical and biochemical observation mandatory in order that the natural history may be fully documented, both in the individual patient and the group as a whole. If patients followed prospectively progress to cirrhosis, then formalised clinical trials of therapy should be considered in patients with sustained abnormalities of liver function tests and biopsy-proven chronic active hepatitis. Such trials have already been started in non-haemophilic patients afflicted with chronic NANB hepatitis and should, over the next 2 years, provide an indication of the agents that might be subjected to controlled evaluation in the haemophilic population. In the meantime, efforts should be continued to eliminate or render non-infective the infective agents in preparations of Factor VIII concentrate.

REFERENCES

1.   Kasper, C.K. and Kipnis, S.A. (1972). Hepatitis and clotting factor concentrates (Letter). J. Am. Med. Assoc., 221, 510

2.   Biggs, R. (1974). Jaundice and antibodies directed against factors VIII and IX in patients treated for haemophilia or Christmas disease in the United Kingdom. Br. J. Haemat., 26, 313

3.   Mannucci, P.M., Capitano, A., Del Ninno, E., Colombo, M., Pareti, M. and Ruggeri, Z.M. (1975). Asymptomatic liver disease in haemophiliacs. J. Clin. Path., 28, 620

4. Levine, P.H., McVerry, B.A., Attock, B. and Dormandy, K. (1977). Health of the intensely treated haemophiliacs, with special reference to abnormal liver chemistries and splenomegaly. Blood, 50, No. 1, 1

5. Bamber, M., Thomas, H.C., and Sherlock, S. (1981). The prevalence of liver dysfunction and hepatitis markers in severe haemophiliacs. (in preparation)

6. Spero, J.A., Lewis, J.H., Van Thiel, D.H., et. al. (1978). Asymptomatic structural liver disease in haemophilia. N. Engl. J. Med., 298, 1373

7. Omata, M., Afroudakis, A., Liew, C., et. al. (1978). Comparison of serum hepatitis B surface antigen (HB_sAg) and serum anti-core antibody (HB_cAb) with tissue HB_sAg and hepatitis B core antigen (HB_cAg). Gastroenterology, 75, 1003

8. Kim, H.C., Said, P., Ackley, A.M., Bringelsen, K.A. and Goche, D.J. (1980). Prevalence of type B and non-A, non-B hepatitis in haemophilia: Relationship to chronic liver disease. Gastroenterology, 79, 1159

9. Knodell, R.G., Conrad, M.E. and Ishak, K.G. (1977). Development of chronic liver disease after acute non-A, non-B post-transfusion hepatitis: Role of gamma globulin prophylaxis in its prevention. Gastroenterology, 72, 902

10. Alter, H.J., Purcell, P.H., Feinstone, S.M., Holland, P.V. and Morrow, A.G. (1978). Non-A, non-B hepatitis: A review and interim report of an ongoing prospective study. In: 'Viral Hepatitis: Etiology, Epidemiology, Pathogenesis and Prevention' (eds.) Vyas, G.N., Cohen, S.N., and Schmid, R. pp. 359-369. (Philadelphia: Franklin Institute Press)

11. Seeff, L.B., Wright, E.C., Zimmerman, H.J., Hoofnagle, J.H., Dietz, A.A., Felsher, B.F., et. al. (1978). Post-transfusion hepatitis, 1973-1975: A Veterans Administration co-operative study. (eds.) Vyas, G.N., Cohen, S.N. and Schmid, R. In: 'Viral Hepatitis: Etiology, Epidemiology, Pathogenesis and Prevention'. pp. 371-381. (Philidelphia: Franklin Institute Press)

34

12. Mosley, J.W., Redeker, A.G., Feinstone, S.M. and Purcell, R.H. (1977). Multiple hepatitis viruses in multiple attacks of acute viral hepatitis. N. Engl. J. Med., 296, 75

13. Tsiquaye, K.N. and Zuckerman, A.J. (1979). New human hepatitis virus. Lancet, i, 1135 (Letter)

14. Shimizu, Y.K., Feinstone, S.M., Alter, H.J. and Purcell R. (1979). Non-A, non-B hepatitis: Ultrastructural alterations associated with acute illness in livers of experimentally infected chimpanzees. Science, 205, 197

15. Tsiquaye, K.N., Bird, R., Tovey, G., Wyke, R.J., Williams, R., and Zuckerman, A.J. (1980). Evidence of cellular changes associated with non-A, non-B hepatitis. J. Med. Virol., 5, 63

16. Myers, T.J., Tembrevilla-Zubiri, C.L., Klatsky, A.U. and Rickles, F.R. (1980). Recurrent acute hepatitis following the use of factor VIII concentrate. Blood, 55, 748

17. Bamber, M., Murray, A.K., Thomas, H.C., Scheuer, P.J., Kernoff, P.B.A. and Sherlock, S. (1981). Clinical and histological features of non-A, non-B hepatitis in a group of patients with congenital coagulation disorders. (Submitted for publication)

18. Craske, J., Dilling, N. and Stern, D. (1975). An outbreak of hepatitis associated with intravenous injection of factor VIII concentrate. Lancet, ii, 221

19. Hruby, M.A. and Schauf, V. (1978). Transfusion-related short-incubation hepatitis in haemophilic patients. J. Am. Med. Assoc., 240, 1355

20. Aach, R.D., Lander, J.J., Sherman, L.A., Miller, W.V., Kahn, R.A., Ghnick, G.L. et. al. (1978). Transfusion-transmitted viruses: Interim analysis of hepatitis among transfused and non-transfused patients. In: (eds.) Vyas, G.N., Cohen, S.N. and Schmid, R. 'Viral Hepatitis: Etiology, Epidemiology, Pathogenesis and Prevention' pp. 383-396 (Philadelphia: Franklin Institute Press)

21. Prince, A.M., Brotman, B., Grady, G.F., Kuhns, W.J., Hazzi, C., Levine, R.W. et. al. (1974). Long-incubation post-transfusion hepatitis without serological evidence of exposure to hepatitis B virus. Lancet, ii, 241

22. Poulsen, H., and Christoffersen, P. (1969). Abnormal bile duct epithelium in liver biopsies with histological signs of viral hepatitis. Acta Path. Microbiol. Scand., 76, 383

23. McVerry, B.A., Voke, J., Mohammed, I., Dormandy, K.M., and Holborrow, E.J. (1977). Immune complexes and abnormal liver function in haemophilia. J. Clin. Pathol., 30, 1142

24. Thomas, H.C., De Villiers, D., Potter, B.J., Hodgson, H., Jain, S., Jewell, D.P. and Sherlock, S. (1978). Immune complexes in acute and chronic liver disease. Clin. Exp. Immunol., 31, 150

25. Thomas, H.C., MacSween, R.N. and White, R.G. (1973). The role of the liver in controlling the immunogenicity of commensal bacteria in the gut. Lancet, i, 1288

26. Prince, A.M., Brotman, B., van den Ende, M.C., Richardson, L. and Kellner, A. (1978). Non-A, non-B hepatitis: Identification of a virus specific antigen and antibody. A preliminary report. In: (eds.) Vyas, G.N., Cohen, S.N. and Schmid, R. 'Viral Hepatitis: Etiology, Epidemiology, Pathogenesis and Prevention'. pp. 633-640. (Philadelphia: Franklin Institute Press)

27. Shirachi, R., Shiraishi, H., Tateda, A., Kikuchi, K. and Ishida, N. (1978). Hepatitis 'C' antigen in non-A, non-B post-transfusion hepatitis. Lancet, ii, 853

28. Vitvitski, L., Trepo, C., Prince, A.M., Brotman, B. (1979). Detection of virus-associated antigen in serum and liver of patients with non-A, non-B hepatitis. Lancet, ii, 1263

29. Feinstone, S.M. and Purcell, R.H. (1978). Non-A, non-B hepatitis. Ann. Rev. Med., 29, 359

30. Bevman, M., Alter, H.J., Ishak, K.G., Purcell, R.H., and Jones,

E.A. (1979). The chronic sequela of non-A, non-B hepatitis. Ann. Int. Med., 91, 1

31. Rakela, J., and Redeker, A. (1979). Chronic liver disease after acute non-A, non-B viral hepatitis. Gastroenterology, 77, 1200

Discussion

Prof. Stewart: You say that you have 10 out of 11 patients with persisting hepatitis, or active hepatitis. Clinically in the non-haemophiliac these are serious conditions, they are progressive, and the patient may eventually die of the disease. What happens in the haemophiliac?

Dr. Thomas: The lesion of chronic active hepatitis, is a progressive lesion, and one would, in a proportion of these patients, expect an element of fibrosis, and ultimately cirrhosis. None of our patients has had cirrhosis, but then, if we are to believe that this illness at the most has been going on since 1974 when the commercial concentrates were first introduced, then this period is short in the course of the disease. There are some indications that these patients may have lesions which will turn to fibrosis or cirrhosis. We have been measuring some of the pro-collagen peptides particularly pro-collagen peptide 3, which is a treated product of pro-collagen after it is altered in the fibroblast. These patients to a man have high levels, three or four times normal and is the sort of level we could expect to see in patients with alcoholic hepatitis who would have a significant risk of going on to develop fibrotic or cirrhotic liver disease. If they maintian these high levels of pro-collagen peptide, they do have a chance of developing fibrosis or cirrhosis ultimately, and the complications that result from that. It is really now a question of how long it takes. Just because we have not seen it in this six-year period, it does not mean that it will not happen. I think the thinking is that it takes ten or twenty years, or even thirty years for these lesions to progress. I think we have to realise that these are young patients, with many years ahead, when we are considering the significance of these lesions. Chronic persistent hepatitis in these patients, from what we know of other groups of such patients, has a much better prognosis, and one would not anticipate that they should come to grief from liver disease.

Dr. Crawford: NHS concentrate has to be made from about 1,000 blood donations, and in general the commercial fractionators decline to broadcast how many donations they use.   Has there been a change since these figures?

Dr. Craske: The actual pool size of the commercial sources is indefinite, I agree, but one should infer, that it is not as large as that currently used for NHS material.   The current size for the large pool NHS concentrate from the Lister Institute is 3,500 donations, and it is likely to decrease.   The point is that the advantage accrued by volunteer donations is probably eliminated by having to use a large pool.   The reason is the amount of plasma per unit from English donations is approximately 200 mls plasma, whereas the advantage of plasmapheresis is that it allows a large amount of plasma to be used from one donor.   The end result of this is that the risk of the large pool NHS concentrate and the commercial concentrate may be similar.

The   other unknown factor is that there is considerable evidence to suggest that the commercial concentrate, particularly that imported from the US, may be associated with a type of non-A, non-B hepatitis which has a low incidence in the U.K.   The other thing I should perhaps like to say is that there is evidence that a small number of haemophiliacs who have come to post-mortem have evidence of having had chronic liver disease, probably contracted years back from long term exposure, acquired in the years before commercial concentrate was ever even thought of, when plasma or cryoprecipitate was used.   No one should take away the idea that commercial concentrate is the sole causative agent.   We must assume that the large pool NHS concentrate is equally involved.

4

Liver biopsy in non-A, non-B hepatitis

P. J. Scheuer

Histological findings are described in six patients with congenital coagulation disorders, who developed hepatitis within 1-4 weeks of receiving factor VIII infusions. Hepatitis A and B infections, Epstein-Barr virus infection and cytomegalovirus hepatitis were excluded serologically. Clinical, biochemical and histological details of the patients are given by Thomas et al.[1]

Two biopsies, taken 1 and 3 months after onset of hepatitis, showed an acute hepatitis. A third, taken at 4 months, showed an excessive portal and periportal inflammatory reaction suggesting possible transition to chronicity. Biopsies taken from two patients 7 and 11 months after onset showed chronic active hepatitis, and in the last patient, also biopsied at 11 months, changes were those of chronic persistent hepatitis. A striking feature in all biopsies except the one taken 1 month after onset was a substantial mononuclear-cell infiltrate in sinusoids, out of proportion to the degree of liver-cell damage. In some specimens this gave an appearance reminiscent of infectious mononucleosis. Damage to bile duct epithelium was seen in three biopsies and was severe in one. Fatty change was seen in both acute and chronic hepatitis.

Pathological changes in this small but apparently homogeneous group of patients with hepatitis were thus distinctive.

REFERENCES

1. Thomas, H.C., Bamber, M., Murray, A., Arborgh, B.A.M., Trepo, C., Scheuer, P.J., Kernoff, P.B.A. and Sherlock, S. Short incubation non-A, non-B hepatitis transmitted by Factor VIII concentrates in patients with congenital coagulation disorders. Submitted for publication.

5

Experience of liver disease in haemophilia

F. E. Preston, D. R. Triger and J. C. E. Underwood

At a meeting of the U.K. Haemophilia Centre Directors a few years ago the view was expressed that slight abnormalities of liver enzymes observed in some haemophilic patients were but a small price to pay when considered against the advantages of modern replacement therapy. Since that time we have been attempting to assess the nature of the liver dysfunction in patients with haemophilia by carrying out a programme of liver biopsy in certain selected patients.

In the first instance we were prompted by two observations which were causing us concern:

1. There appeared to be an extremely high incidence of abnormal liver function test in our regularly treated haemophiliacs.

2. The increasing frequency of acute hepatitis in our haemophilic population.

Standard liver function tests were performed routinely on 87 patients in the Sheffield Haemophilia Centre. Abnormalities in one or more liver function tests have been found in 76 (88%); the nature of these are shown in Table 1. Frequently these are transient but those with persistent abnormality in tests for more than 6 months have been considered for liver biopsy[1,2].

Despite the high incidence of abnormal biochemical tests, only one patient had any persistent symptoms referable to the liver (a patient who had had clinical hepatitis 18 months previously and who suffered recurrent bouts of abdominal pain). 30% of all patients gave a history consistent with an episode of hepatitis at some time in the past. Apart from hepatomegaly (two patients) and palpable splenomegaly (one patient) there were no abnormal physical signs on examination.

Table 1   Incidence of abnormal liver function tests in 87 Sheffield haemophilia patients

Elevated bilirubin	34%
Elevated alkaline phosphatase*	23%
Elevated SGOT	64% — Severe haemophiliacs 86%
Elevated SGPT	78% — Mild haemophiliacs 74%
No abnormality	12%

*5-Nucleotidase in children

Serological markers of hepatitis B virus (HBV) infection were examined in all patients. Persistent $HB_s Ag$ by radioimmunoassay (RIA) was detected in only one patient, but anti-HB_s (RIA) was found in 46 (54%) and anti-HB_c by immunoelectrophoresis in 60 (69%). No HBV markers were detected in only 18 patients.

LIVER BIOPSY

Before each liver biopsy, the presence of Factor VIII inhibitors was excluded and a calculated dose of Factor VIII concentrate was given sufficient to elevate the patient's Factor VIII level to 1.0 U/ml. With regular monitoring and further administrations of Factor VIII this level was maintained above 0.5 U/ml for the next 72 hours. One patient with von Willebrand's disease was given DDAVP, the vasopressin analogue. In this patient Factor VIII levels were also maintained above 0.5 U/ml for 72 hours after the liver biopsy.

LIVER BIOPSY RESULTS

We have now examined liver biopsies from 19 haemophiliacs, including 5 children whose ages range from 2 to 10 years, and one patient with von Willebrand's disease. Nineteen of these were percutaneous needle biopsies, one was a wedge biopsy taken at laparotomy from a haemophiliac with Hodgkin's disease. The morphological diagnoses are shown in Table 2.

Table 2   Spectrum of liver disease in biopsies from 20 haemophiliacs

Morphological diagnosis*	Number of patients	
Acute hepatitis	0	
CPH	12	
CPH/CAH borderline	2	
Mild/moderate CAH	4)	
Severe CAH	1)	cirrhosis 3
Non-specific reactive hepatitis	1)	

* CPH = chronic persistent hepatitis
  CAH = chronic active (aggressive) hepatitis

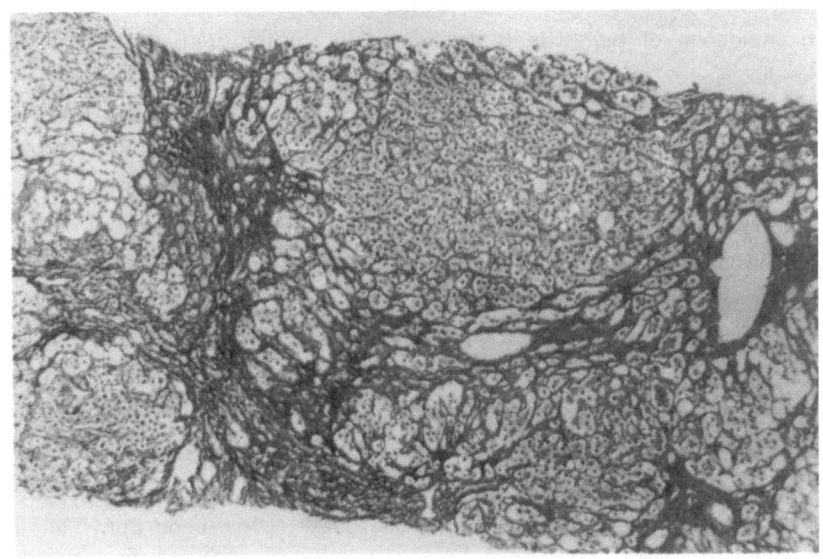

Figure 1   Cirrhosis arising in severe chronic active (aggressive) hepatitis in a haemophiliac. Fibrous septae disrupt the lobular architecture. Reticulin stain x 50

The biopsy findings ranged from chronic persistent hepatitis, present in the majority of our cases, to severe chronic active (aggressive) hepatitis with evolving or established cirrhosis (Figure 1). Unexplained granulomas were an additional feature in two biopsies. Non-specific reactive hepatitis was present in the wedge biopsy from our patient with Hodgkin's disease.

All of the biopsies were further examined by electron microscopy. No specific features were noted and no virus particles were found.

CLINICAL SIGNIFICANCE OF BIOPSY FINDINGS

Chronic persistent hepatitis is typically a benign disorder that rarely proceeds to cirrhosis, whereas chronic active (aggressive) hepatitis carries a significant risk of progression to cirrhosis and sometimes merits treatment with steroids. Haemophiliacs are, however, repeatedly exposed to hepatitis virus or viruses and we do not yet know what effect this may have on the course of chronic liver disease in these patients.

In our series, there was no correlation between the biochemical abnormalities and the histological diagnosis on liver biopsy. Despite the high incidence of hepatitis B markers, the contribution of HBV to chronic liver disease in haemophiliacs is debatable. Two out of 15 adults and 4 out of 5 children with histological evidence of chronic liver disease had no HBV markers. Most of the children have only received Factor VIII replacement therapy since the introduction of hepatitis B screening of all donors by RIA. This raises the possibility of non-A, non-B viruses as aetiological agents in chronic hepatitis in haemophiliacs.

COMPLICATIONS

Only two complications attributable to the procedure have been encountered in our patients. A 9 year old boy with severe chronic active (aggressive) hepatitis was re-admitted to hospital 5 days after the biopsy with abdominal pain, jaundice and melaena. Ultrasonography showed an enlarged gall bladder thought to be full of blood and a clinical diagnosis of haemobilia was made. The patient was treated with Factor VIII alone and made an uneventful recovery. There have been no further complications in 2 years follow-up. A 50 year old man developed HB_sAg positive hepatitis 3 months after his liver biopsy. This was attributed to the concentrate used to cover the procedure because another haemophiliac also acquired hepatitis B in relation to the same batch of concentrate given for a joint bleed. Six month follow-up has shown that this patient with chronic persistent hepatitis has cleared the hepatitis B antigen, recovered clinically from hepatitis and his biochemical abnormalitites are now similar to those prior to biopsy.

CONCLUSIONS

1. Liver biopsy may be performed in haemophiliac patients with a low incidence of complications.

2. There is a high incidence of chronic liver disease in treated haemophiliac patients, the nature of which is not predictable by standard liver function tests.

3. Neither symptoms nor signs are a reliable guide to the presence or severity of liver disease in these patients.

4. Non-A, non-B hepatitis viruses are likely to be at least as important in the pathogenesis of the liver disease as hepatitis B.

REFERENCES

1. Preston, F.E., Triger, D.R., Underwood, J.C.E., Bardhan, G., Steward, R.M. and Blackburn, E.K. (1978). Percutaneous liver biopsy and chronic liver disease in haemophiliacs. Lancet, 2, 592

2. McGrath, K.M., Lilleyman, J.S., Triger, D.R. and Underwood, J.C.E. (1980). Liver disease complicating severe haemophilia in childhood. Arch. Dis. Child., 55, 537

Discussion

Prof. Scheuer: I wanted to ask about the transaminases in your patients. Professor Sherlock has noted in the non-B post-transfusion hepatitis patients there is a very striking fluctuation of transaminases, and she says she can look at the transaminase chart and guess that the patient has non-A, non-B. Do you find that?

Dr. Triger: We probably have selected out ones that would not be covered by that statement, because we have tended to take people that have been consistently abnormal, and the ones that have gone back to normal we have not biopsied. In fact, most of ours have consistently elevated enzymes. Either they have been found to be twice normal or so, or in the case of the von Willebrand's patients they have been 8 to 10 times normal each time we have tested them, over a period of two years or more. So it has not been our limited experience.

Dr. Underwood: In the patients that we have followed serially for at least two years, the pattern had been fluctuating to begin with, and then there was a tendency as the peak levels came down to reach a plateau. In 2 or 3 patients with longer follow up we have seen a transition from the fluctuating to a more persistent abnormality, so it might be a feature of the early phase of the disease. In a one-point-in-time study without a defined onset one would be coming in later, and that would fit with the more severe histology in Prof. Scheuer's patients than in ours. We are looking at the first 2 to 3 years of the illness, and he is looking at anything up to 6 years after the onset, assuming it was related to the change in practice of administration of Factor VIII concentrates in 1974.

Prof. Scheuer: I think that is right, and in the 5 children in whom we can date the maximum length of exposure, but have no history of hepatitis, we have an arbitrary starting point. This has not been a notable feature in the ones we have noted. But I accept your interpretation.

Dr. Craske: That is an interesting observation about the fluctuations because we have found in 2 groups of haemophiliacs that we have looked at for abnormal liver function tests, about 30 per cent of them have one abnormal test and then we test them again frequently and find them normal. This may reflect cases where by sampling more often we find the pattern that Dr. Thomas has suggested.

Prof. Bloom: Could the appropriate members of the panel advise the Haemophilia Centres Directors and the clinicians who are present, on what is the current state regarding the possible treatment of these various types of hepatitis?   Should we be doing liver biopsies in practice on our haemophiliacs, and if we do, can we correlate possible treatment to the liver biopsy appearances?

Dr. Thomas: I would like to answer this in two parts.   At the moment we are at a stage of observing what the spectrum of inflammatory lesions is in these patients.   I would suggest that we are at a stage now where we have got an idea of the sorts of lesions that we are seeing.   A significant proportion, perhaps 40 or 50 per cent, have chronic active hepatitis.   Prof. Scheuer pointed out that we can only speculate on the course that this inflammatory lesion will have in this particular group of patients, and draw analogies to hepatitis-B, chronic active hepatitis, and the auto-immune form of chronic active hepatitis.   It is much more likely that this form, since it is presumed to be caused by a virus, will be more closely analogous to the hepatitis-B form of chronic active hepatitis, and that group has not shown benefit from receiving immuno-suppressant therapy, although it would be wrong to assume that this other form of virus-induced liver disease will behave in the same way.   It might be possible to consider some form of trial of therapy.

An alternative approach is to observe them for longer and to try and ascertain the natural history of this group of patients.   My own feeling is based primarily on two facts.   We are studying the patients fairly early on, perhaps 2 years or so at the maximum after onset of illness, and we are not seeing much in the way of fibrosis, whereas Dr. Triger is studying it perhaps a few years further on and he has got a significant incident of cirrhosis. So it may be a progressive lesion.

The second reason for feeling that it might be progressive is that we have been looking at the pro-collagen peptides, particularly the pro-collagen 3, in these patients, and this is a measure of collagen synthesis. If the increased levels that we are seeing in these patients continue, one would predict that they would get fibrotic liver disease and the complications that go along with that.

One can predict that there will be problems in the future. The issue that we have to decide is whether we should start trials to see whether we could do anything about that, or whether we should follow these patients for longer to see if this predictive natural history is indeed so.

Dr. Triger: · I would agree with what Dr. Thomas said. Perhaps I can add an ancedote. We were faced with this problem 3 years ago, when we uncovered a case of non-A, non-B hepatitis with a chronic aggressive picture in a young man in his twenties. We decided that we would try to treat him with corticosteroids. We have done this for years now. I got out his serial tests and there is really no convincing evidence that he had improved or responded on steroids. It looked like it for the first 6 months, but when we take the whole picture it does not look like it.

However, enzymes are one thing; histology is another. I know that my colleagues will agree with me that we really need histological backing, not only on Day 1, the static study, but really to see what happens over several years. We are planning, with this man's agreement, to repeat the liver biopsy very shortly, and to biopsy 2 or 3 others that we have biopsied in the past and in whom there is genuine doubt as to what is happening with the liver.

Prof. Scheuer: The American literature on post-transfusion hepatitis has suggested that compared to the B virus, the non-A, non-B tends to be more symptomless. Secondly, the incidence of serious sequelae is likely to be higher than the B. Is there any evidence from patients that would support these conclusions and was the concentrate used in the two centres of American origin or European?

Dr. Thomas: Before commenting, we must answer the issue as to whether the hepatitis that we are seeing in the concentrate-infused patients is the same as the post-transfusion hepatitis. My own belief, and Prof. Scheuer's and Prof. Zuckerman's on the basis of his chimpanzee studies, is that it might be a different virus, although we have yet to produce serological proof of that. If it is a different virus, then we cannot conclude too much from the course of the post-transfusion non-A, non-B hepatitis. The course of that post-transfusion hepatitis has tended to be one of improvement with the course of the illness. In a study from NIH, the transaminase levels tended to come down, as we have seen, and the impression was that over 2 or 3 years the lesions tended to improve. I know that in a post-plasmapheresis non-A, non-B hepatitis of the 7 to 10 week incubation type, when the patients were biopsied they had a very mild lesion, chronic persistent hepatitis, and no increased levels of pro-collagen peptides, so they had no evidence of progressive fibrosis. I think that this form probably does have a benign course, and I think that the short incubation type, for want of a better term, in the haemophiliac patients appears to be something different, and it remains to be seen what course that takes. The prediction is that it will be a more significiant progressive illness, and I think they will develop fibrosis. Indeed, Dr. Triger's studies have shown that a significant proportion have cirrhosis.

I can say something about the Royal Free patients. They received mostly commercial concentrate. Always a brand that they had received before and often a batch that they had recently received.

Prof. Scheuer: As far as the 6 patients whose biopsies I showed are concerned, 2 or 3 of them were still in the acute phase, but all of them showed biochemical and chemical chronicity, although none of them has been re-biopsied so far. In that particular series, the chronicity appears to be 100 per cent. What the implication is for cirrhosis we have no idea.

Anonymous: Is there any evidence that continuing antigenic stimulus, either in haemophilia or in any other hepatitis situation means that things are likely to get worse or better?

Dr. Thomas: I do not think we know in respect of continuing exposure to the virus. There is some information from Dr. Popper's early studies where he was injecting bovine protein into rats, and in those animals which produced an immune response to the porcine proteins – there was development of portal fibrosis, presumably on the basis of immune complex formation and deposition in these areas. In that context, if the Factor VIII concentrates are at least partially immunogenic because of denaturation of some of the proteins, then this sort of phenomenon might be superimposed. We looked at one patient in the early phases of our studies with Dr. Kernoff. Because of the suggestion that it might be a response to a foreign protein, we thought we might see immune complex formation and complement activation products. We followed one patient very carefully immediately before and during and after the infusion, and showed no evidence of such a phenomenon, although we have not really done extensive studies.

Prof. Stewart: Have the effects of continued infection been taken into account in the study of these biopsies, and in the effect of therapy?

Dr. Thomas: Some patients have had repeated infusions. Three patients have had just a single infusion, and this remitting course, particularly in respect of the transaminases was seen equally obviously in the 3 who have had just a single infusion, as in those that had subsequently received further infusions. It did not appear to influence this rather fluctuating course, although the numbers involved are relatively small, and it is still possible.

Prof. MacSween: Has evidence of glomerular nephritis been sought in these patients?

Dr. Thomas: No.

Dr. Triger: We have not gone so far as to do renal biopsies on any of them, but we have certainly looked for proteinuria and for cell sediment, and we have not seen any evidence.

Prof. Scheuer: If I could add a further comment to what Dr. Thomas was mentioning earlier about the chimpanzee experiment. I think we could go a bit further now and say that in all our experiments so far, we feel quite clearly that there are two agents present in different factors that we have found both from UK and European sources, and also in the United States, and there are a couple of papers in press that put together a lot of the chimpanzee transmission data with these different materials. I would also add that although we are still calling these short and long-incubation and non-A, non-B hepatitis, I think that is one area where there is considerable debate - how exactly these incubation periods define these two types of agents. But on biological grounds at least in cross challenge experiments on chimps, it looks quite clear that there are at least two different agents.

Prof. MacSween: Following on from that, I should like to ask Prof. Scheuer if he knows whether any other group has looked at biopsies from their cases, in which there is a definable antigen-antibody system and characteristic electron microscopic appearances. Do they histologically resemble those that he has seen?

Prof. Scheuer: I do not yet know. I have not seen them. I am rather looking forward to seeing them.

Dr. Thomas: I think the general impression - just by word of mouth -is that they are milder in terms of the amount of lobular hepatitis. Similarly the cases in the German plasmapheresis studies have been much milder, tending towards chronic persistence, or at the most a borderline chronic active, not this lobular infiltrate that Prof. Scheuer has shown.

Prof. Steward: Presumably the suggestion is that this comes from the blood, that this is a viral particle. Surely this should be detectable in some patients receiving multiple transfusions. Everything has been blamed on to concentrates so far, but surely this should be detectable in other patients who have received much transfusion.

Prof. MacSween: One would anticipate the reply by saying that the basis for the existence of a non-A, non-B came from the failure of screening of donors for hepatitis B - the failure of that to prevent post-transfusion hepatitis in patients who were getting whole blood. It then became evident in those who were getting concentrates that the incidence of abnormal liver function tests in these patients was considerably higher, and was presumably in part dose related. That is my simplistic assessment of it.

Dr. Thomas: Yes. I think we should view hepatitis B infection as the odd man out, and we are lulled into a rather secure feeling by the fact that the viral antigens can be detected in the serum of the HBV infected patient. Really non-A, non-B is running more akin to other infections in that it is very difficult to detect virus in the blood. I think there have been some titration studies, particularly by Purcell's group, showing that the number of infectious units in a ml of blood is several logs less in respect of the non-A, non-B viruses when compared to hepatitis B - i.e. there is much less virus there. Some Japanese workers have cited a virus-like particle, but that is subjudice at the moment, and it remains to be seen whether other people come up with the same morphological particle.

Prof. Stewart: The chance is that these patients are receiving a whole unit, so even a small amount of virus particle would be a lot. If it is assumed that this is a comparatively uncommon contaminant in the blood, which because of the larger pool size of fractions is present, therefore, in an effective concentration in concentrates, one would expect somewhere along the line to see patients who received a large dose who are much worse off.

Dr. Craske: Part of the answer to Prof. Stewart's question lies in the different prevalence of non-A, non-B hepatitis in America, where they perhaps know more about the question than anywhere else. I am certain that one estimate of the number of carriers, made at a meeting I was at recently, was that of the order of 5 per cent of donors might be carriers of non-A, non-B virus in some populations. This is certainly not the case in the UK when the actual incidence of reported non-A, non-B hepatitis after whole blood transfusions is very low, and the only two instances I know of, 2 or 3 cases in a year, which is equivalent to the sort of level one gets with hepatitis B in a donor screened population. So I think we are dealing with a different order of non-A, non-B hepatitis in the English population. The reason why one sees a comparable incidence of non-A, non-B hepatitis after NHS Factor VIII is the large pool size we have to use because of the small unit of plasma from each donation. I think that is something that has to be borne in mind.

Dr. Steven: Can I ask the London and Sheffied clinicans respectively what, if any, precautions they take when handling the blood and liver samples from these patients.

Prof. Scheuer: I take exactly the same precautions, or lack of precautions that I do with all my patients with liver disease or suspected liver disease. Anybody who may have liver disease may have a potentially infectious source, but it is not horrifically infectious and it is to be treated with respect. I do not really treat them with more or less respect than any other high-risk hospital group of patients.

Dr. Triger: We have the same approach. I think we accord them the same care as we do with any other liver patient. I think a little less than we do with the HBV infected patients at the moment, although that is not perhaps a very justifiable position to take. Once again - where there have been titrations of the number of infective units within a unit of plasma, there is a much lower level of virus in the non-A, non-B situation than compared with the B. It may be that a larger volume of blood is therefore needed to transmit an infective dose. But we do not know that yet.

Dr. Craske: There are well-documented needle sticker cases of non-A, non-B as well as B.

Dr. Jones: Could we come back and try to put this into perspective. One of the speakers quite rightly said that yes, we see abnormal function tests, yes we obviously see abnormal biopsy. Patients in the UK have now been chronically transfused with commercial concentrate for over 7 years, and in the US and Germany for considerably longer at considerably higher doses. What we do not seem to have seen is chronic morbidity or increasing mortality from liver disease. I wonder if we should be seeing that in the UK now, and if any of the Americans present might care to comment on that.

Prof. MacSween: That seems a logical sequence to follow on the preliminary studies - is there evidence of an increased morbidity as a result of this?

Dr. Triger: We certainly do not have anything very much in the way of obvious morbidity without looking. We are dealing with chronic liver disease, in which 5 to 7 years is a very short time - as we all know. 10 to 20 years may be a long time, but we have been looking at liver biopsies of children under the age of 10 years, and what we are concerned with is what is likely to happen to them when they should be fit, healthy 25 year olds. I was shown in Pittsburgh two horrendous cases of 18 and 21 year olds with large, juicy oesophageal varices, that the physician just hopes he is in Europe when they burst, because he does not know what he will do, I think we are just building up trouble.

Dr. Thomas: I think our view is the same. If we draw the analogy to hepatitis B infection, many of these patients are infected at birth, at least in Africa. They do not get problems till the third decade of life. One might reasonably justify an analogy to that sort of infection. As Dr. Triger has said, it is in 10 years time that we shall see the problems. Bearing in mind the proportion of the patients that are infected, or have persistent abnormal liver function tests, anything from 60 to 80 per cent, it will be an enormous problem when it happens.

6

The development of hepatitis B vaccines and antiviral therapy

C. R. Howard

Hepatitis B is presently a major public health problem with an estimated 175 million persistently infected carriers throughout the world. Acute or chronic hepatitis infection is manifested by the expression of several gene products, the surface antigen (HB_sAg) being particularly abundant in blood and serum as 22nm spherical particles. Active virus replication additionally gives rise to detectable numbers of double-shelled particles containing an antigenically distinct core component (HB_cAg) within which the viral DNA genome is encapsidated. Hepatitis B e antigen (HB_eAg) is a third, immunologically distinct marker of active virus replication which exists predominantly as a molecular entity separate from the 22nm HB_sAg particles and may be released from the core of complete virus particles by detergent treatment. The properties and diagnostic features of hepatitis B antigens have recently been reviewed[1].

A hepatitis B vaccine is urgently required for the protection of groups at high risk of acquiring the infection. These groups include individuals requiring repeated transfusions of blood or blood products, prolonged in-patient care, patients who require frequent tissue penetration or who have natural or acquired immune deficiency and those persons with malignant diseases. Viral hepatitis is also a major occupational hazard among staff of haemodialysis units and institutions for the mentally retarded and among dental surgeons. In addition, high rates of infection occur in drug addicts, homosexuals and prostitutes. In certain areas of the world, the high carriage rate of HBV is most probably maintained by the maternal transmission of virus to neonates; the availability of a hepatitis B vaccine is therefore also desirable for the effective reduction of the numbers persistently infected with this virus.

Active Immunisation Against Hepatitis B

Early attempts to vaccinate against hepatitis B using infectious serum heated at 98°C for 1 minute prevented or modified hepatitis B in 69% of 29 volunteers subsequently challenged with the original infectious serum 4-8 months later[2,3]. The results were essentially the same after one, two or three inoculations and established that serum from individuals infected with hepatitis B virus (HBV) could be used as a source of viral antigens for inducing a protective immune response. Soulier and colleagues[4] used HB_sAg serum from a persistently infected donor heated at 60°C for 10 hours but the virus was not effectively inactivated as shown by the development of HB_sAg accompanied by raised ALT levels in some of the recipients. Electron microscopy has shown that such sera contain both complete HBV particles and numerous 22 nm HB_sAg particles (Figure 1). In the absence of conventional tissue culture systems for the in vitro growth of HBV, plasma collected from large numbers of infected blood donors is the major source of virus-containing material for vaccine development.

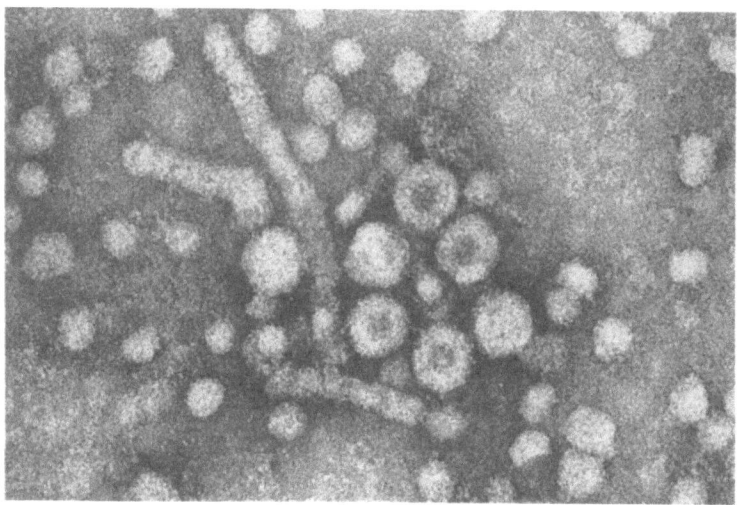

Figure 1   Negative staining microscopy of hepatitis B antigen. Small 22 nm HBsAg spherical particles and filaments are abundant in the sera of infected individuals. The hepatitis B virus is occasionally seen in a larger 42 nm articles with a distinct 27 nm core

Human HBV has been successfully transmitted to chimpanzees and although the infection is generally mild, the biochemical, histological and serological responses in these primates are very similar to those in humans and antigenic markers of virus replication are antigenically indistinguishable from the homologous antigens and antibodies from man. Chimpanzees therefore, offer an ideal experimental model for the evaluation of experimental hepatitis B vaccines. Vaccines prepared from the 22 nm HB_sAg particles after purification from plasma and inactivation by formaldehyde have been shown to be safe and protective in susceptible primates, leading to the production of antibody to HB_sAg[5,6] (Figure 2).

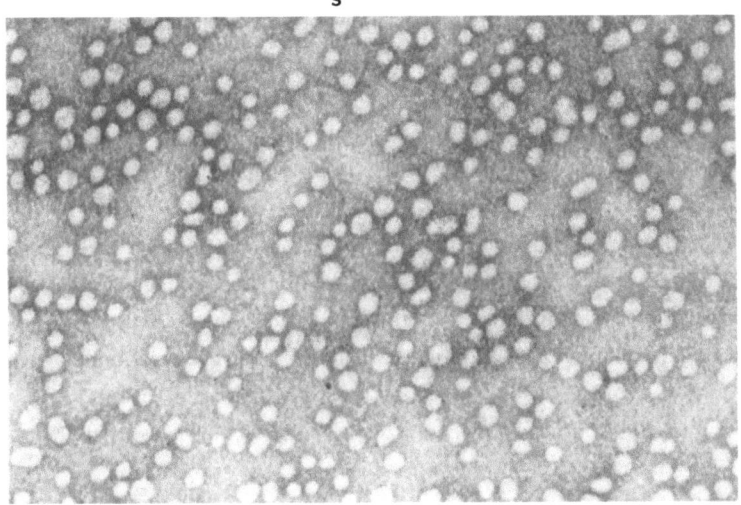

Figure 2   Purified preparation of 22 nm HBsAg particles. Similar preparations are currently under investigation as suitable vaccines for the immunoprophylaxis of hepatitis B

The use of a vaccine derived from infected individuals represents a major departure from conventional approaches to preventive medicine. The World Health Organisation Expert Committee on Viral Hepatitis has therefore proposed guidelines and criteria for the safe development of hepatitis B vaccines. The more important points may be listed as follows:

1. HB_sAg-positive blood donations selected for the preparation of a vaccine should be devoid of HBV as assessed by the absence of virus-associated DNA polymerase activity and HB_eAg. The absence of these markers is associated with a lower risk of infectivity, although the association is not absolute. In addition, such sera invariably possess smaller quantities of HB_sAg thereby increasing the volume of starting material required.

2.   Preparation procedures should be designed to remove most, if not all, contaminants, especially complete HBV particles.

3.   Final vaccine preparations should be treated by accepted inactivation

procedures. The use of formaldehyde is currently favoured for the inactivation of residual HBV or any other adventitious agents.

4.   The absence of infectious HBV must be confirmed by appropriate safety tests in non-immune chimpanzees.

5.   The preparative procedure should yield a vaccine that is immunogenic and capable of protecting against challenge with live HBV in chimpanzees.

Other considerations include minimising the risk that agents of non-A, non-B are present by the repeated use of a relatively small number of donors and careful design of clinical trials for the evaluation of hepatitis B vaccines in man. The Expert Committee has recommended that the safety of any vaccine preparation must be demonstrated in a small group of healthy adult volunteers before administration to a larger group. The long term follow-up of recipients is regarded as an essential criterion in the development of hepatitis B immunoprophylaxis, with careful monitoring of specifc anti-HB_s levels and frequent examination for non-specific immune responses to contaminating antigens, development of hepatitis and the presence of autoimmune markers.

The first human trial using partially pure 22 nm HB_sAg preparations was reported by Maupas and colleagues[7] who administered vaccine to the patients and staff of several haemodialysis units in France. Although this study did not include a control group, there was subsequently a significant difference in the incidence of hepatitis B infection between the immunised group and a group of patients and staff who had not received the vaccine. Hilleman et al.[8] conducted a small trial in volunteers using a purified 22 nm preparation treated with formaldehyde. This vaccine had previously been shown to protect chimpanzees against challenge with HBV. Volunteers received the vaccine in either aqueous form. or with an alum adjuvant; in both groups the preparation elicited antibody to HB_sAg in individuals with and without pre-existing homologous antibody. Carefully controlled field trials using similar preparations are now in progress in the USA and include various groups at high risk such as patients and staff of haemodialysis units and young male homosexuals[9].

The Development of "Second Generation" Hepatitis B Vaccines

Biochemical analyses have repeatedly shown that the 22 nm HB_sAg

particle is a complex structure consisting of lipid and several proteins of either host or viral origin. In particular, a close association between human serum albumin and the 22 nm particle has been established[10]. Hepatitis B-specific antigenic determinants are associated with an unglycosylated polypeptide with a molecular weight in the range of 22-24,000 and a glycosylated polypeptide with a molecular weight in the range of 26-29,000[1]. Both polypeptides may exist as a 49,000 molecular weight complex under non-reducing conditions[11], and have identical amino acid sequences at amino acid carboxyl terminals, indicating that the larger polypeptide represents a glycosylated form of the smaller non-glycosylated polypeptide[12]. Although the 22 nm HB_sAg particles share a common antigen with the outer coat of the HBV particle, there exists the possibility that the presence of host proteins, in particular serum albumin, might either depress the level and intensity of the anti-HB_s response or induce undesirable immunological side reactions. In anticipation of a successful outcome of clinical trials using intact 22 nm HB_sAg particles, several approaches are being considered for the formulation of hepatitis B vaccines which exclusively contain virus-specific material. It is considered that vaccines prepared from the constituent polypeptides of HB_sAg would have an added margin of safety since the preparations would be chemically well-defined and even less likely to contain contaminating virus or host components.

Solubilisation of the integral proteins of the 22 nm particles may be readily accomplished by disruption of the lipid bilayer with non-ionic detergents such as Triton X-100. In general, the biological and antigenic properties of viral proteins are preserved in contrast to the use of strongly ionic detergents. Both virus-specific polypeptides can be extracted as a 3.9S complex from intact HB_sAg 22 nm particles by Triton X-100 solubilisation and affinity chromatography on concanavalin A-Sepharose with retention of antigenic activity[10]. Monomeric solutions of polypeptides in detergent are poor immunogens, and therefore unsuitable for use as vaccines. Recently, a method of removal of Triton X-100 from solubilised membrane polypeptides was developed, whereby the polypeptides are sedimented into a detergent-free sucrose gradient under defined conditions, resulting in the formation of polypeptide micelles[13]. These structures are water soluble by virtue of the fact that hydrophilic residues are exposed to the aqueous environment and the hydrophobic portions of the polypeptides are sequestered in the interior of the particle. Solubilised HB_sAg polypeptides treated by this procedure consistenly formed micellar structures with an average diameter of 120 nm[14]. The buoyant density of the HB_sAg micelles

60

was 1.25 g/m. as compared with 1.19 g/ml for the original intact particle, an increase consistent with the removal of most of the lipid by the solubilisation procedure. The two component polypeptides of the micelles were present in the same stoichiometric ratio as in the original Triton X-100 solubilised HB_sAg fraction and the antigenic activity of the HB_sAg polypeptides was preserved throughout the process of solubilisation and reassociation.

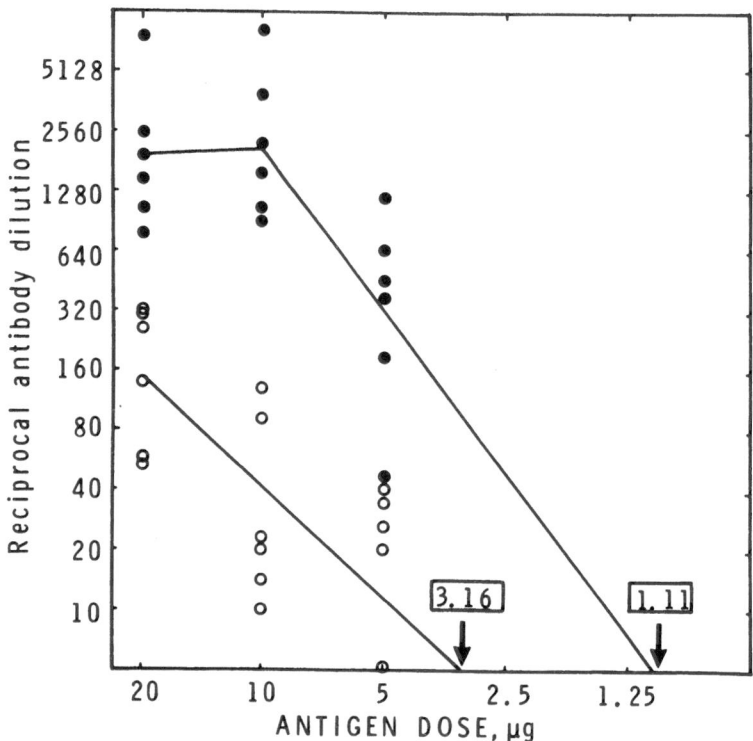

Figure 3   Geometric mean antibody titres at differing dose levels of either HBsAg 22 nm particles (o) or HBsAg micelles (o). Each point represents the titre in a single animal. The antigen extinction doses in each case are indicated (taken from ref. 14)

The immunogenicity of the HB_sAg micelles has been compared with that of intact HB_sAg 22 nm particles by inoculation of SWR/J strain mice in the presence of an alum adjuvant. It has been suggested that the serological response in mice may be a useful indicator of the immunogenic potential of candidate hepatitis B vaccines[15]. Three doses of alum-adjuvanted preparations were tested in three groups of animals respectively. In each group, the titre of anti-HB_s induced by the micelles greatly exceeded that induced by intact 22 nm particles (Figure 3). Furthermore, the slopes of the dilution curves obtained by radioimmunoassy indicated an enhanced antibody affinity in the sera of mice receiving HB_sAg micelles.

The high surface antibody titres induced by HB_sAg micelles may be due to one or more interacting factors. These factors include the larger size of the micelles, altered distribution of antigenic sites, and the absence in the micelles of serum albumin and other host-derived proteins, which may, singularly or in combination, affect the nature of the antibody response. In the case of influenza, for example, the relative potency of "split" vaccine compared to the whole inactivated virus has been found to be dependent on the presence or absence of adjuvant[15]. In an animal model HB_sAg polypeptide micelles were better immunogens than intact HB_sAg using an adjuvant suitable for human use. The chemical purity, specific serological activity and powerful immunogenicity of the micelles, taken together with ease of preparation on a large scale, strongly favour their development as an alternative "second-generation" hepatitis B vaccine. This physical form may indeed also be suitable for vaccines prepared using HB_sAg polypeptides produced by the expression of cloned hepatitis B virus DNA and E. coli or other hosts[17]. Experiments to test the immunogenicity, safety and protective capacity of HB_sAg micelles in primates and in man are currently in progress.

Antiviral Therapy of Chronic Hepatitis B
Interferon

Several studies have indicated that the administration of human interferon both in humans and chimpanzees has an inhibitory effect on ongoing hepatitis B virus replication. In an early study, transient changes in markers of virus activity were observed when leucocyte interferon was given for less then 2 weeks, although more prolonged treatment of 2 patients with chronic active hepatitis resulted in a marked drop in the number of circulating virus particles which persisted for up to 15 weeks after stopping treatment[18]. A more extensive study of the use of leucocyte interferon was reported by Scullard and colleagues[19], who treated 8 patients with chronic hepatitis B for periods of 5-8 weeks and in one case for 5 months. In one patient, there was a marked fall in the number of virus particles in the blood which coincided with the disappearance of HB_eAg and a reduction in aspartate aminotransferase levels. In three other patients, a similar effect was seen but proved to be transient, whereas in a fourth hepatitis B-associated DNA polymerase activity continued to rise despite treatment. Although there was no significant change in HB_sAg titres in these patients, a marked decrease in cytotoxic T-cell activity towards HB_sAg-coated target cells was found. This important observation suggests that the antiviral effect of leucocyte interferon may be offset by a depression of cell-mediated responses to infected hepatocytes, resulting in impaired clearance of the virus despite a reduction in the extent of hepatitis B virus replication. Persistently infected female patients appear to respond better to interferon, as noted by Scullard et al. and a similar study reported by Merigan and Robinson[20].

Similar results using fibroblast interferon have also been reported [20,21], although interferon produced by fibroblasts appears to be somewhat less potent: in one study, a 2 week course of treatment with interferon from human fibroblasts failed to produce any significant changes in markers of hepatitis B virus replication.

Leucocyte interferon has been shown to be considerably more immunosuppressive than fibroblast interferon[29], augmenting natural killer cell activity[30,31]. At present, there is a noticeable lack of information regarding the relative level of circulating interferon in actue and chronically infected patients: the interferon-natural killer cell system may be of paramount importance in recovery from acute disease with persistent virus arising as a result of a deficiency in either interferon production or natural killer cell activity[32].

Ribavirin (1-β-D-ribofuranosyl-1,2,4,-triazole-3-carboxamide)
Ribavirin, also known as Virazole, is a synthetic nucleoside analogue with a broad spectrum of antiviral activity against viruses with both RNA and DNA genomes. The phosphorylated derivative is a competitive inhibitor of IMP dehydrogenase, an intracellular enzyme required in GMP biosynthesis. Ribavirin may be administered orally to patients in a dose of 800 mg daily for a month without evidence of toxicity, and is licensed for use in several countries.

Early studies involving acute hepatitis B patients in South America as well as in persistent carriers of HB_sAg were encouraging[23,24]. However, no significant changes in hepatitis B markers were found in persistently infected chimpanzees treated with the drug[25,26].

Ara-A

Ara-A is an analogue of the adenine deoxyribonucleoside, and in contrast to other pyrimidine analogues is virtually non-toxic, being rapidly de-aminated in vivo and converted to hypoxanthine arabinoside. The antiviral activity of ara-A in the treatment of herpes infections has been well documented. The treatment of chronic active hepatitis B in two patients was reported by Pollard et al.[27]. Both received two courses of treatment for up to 2 weeks each. In one patient there was a rapid decrease in the level of hepatitis B-associated DNA polymerase activity during both courses of treatment, although a return to pre-treatment levels was seen during the 7 week period between courses and after cessation of the second course. In the second patient, the reduction in DNA polymerase activity was more prolonged, the second course resulting in a reduction in DNA polymerase activity to an undetectable level which persisted 12 months beyond the treatment period. Chadwick et al.[28] using a single, shorter course of treatment found that the effects of ara-A were transient in 3 of 4 patients with chronic liver disease treated with the drug. A reduction in HB_sAg titre was seen in the fourth patient who was negative for specific DHA polymerase activity. Merigan and Robinson[20] also found a variable response after ara-A treatment: although circulating virus was reduced during treatment in all 4 patients studied, in 2 these changes did not persist. Similar temporary effects in persistently infected chimpanzees treated with ara-A were reported by Zuckerman et al.[26]. It remains to be established whether continued treatment with this drug above, or in a phosphorylated form, or in combination with interferon, will have a more lasting effect on hepatitis B virus replication.

REFERENCES

1.   Zuckerman, A.J. and Howard, C.R. (1979). Hepatitis Viruses of Man (London: Academic Press)

2.   Krugman, S., Giles, J.P. and Hammond, J. (1971). Viral hepatitis type B (MS-2 strain). Studies on active immunisation. J. Am. Med. Assoc., 217, 41

3.   Krugman, S. and Giles, J.P. (1973). Viral hepatitis type B (MS-2 strain). Further observations on natural history and prevention. N. Engl. J. Med., 288, 755

4. Soulier, J.P., Blatix, C., Courouce, A.M., Benamon, D., Amouch, P. and Drouvet, J. (1972). Prevention of virus B hepatitis (SH hepatitis). Am. J. Dis. Child., 123, 429

5. Buynak, E.B., Roehm, R.R., Tylell, A.A., Bertland, A.U., Lampson, G.P. and Hilleman, M.R. (1976). Vaccine against human hepatitis B. J. Am. Med. Assoc., 235, 2832

6. Purcell, R.H. and Gerin, J.L. (1978). Hepatitis B vaccines: a status report. In: G.N. Vyas, S.N. Cohen and R. Schmid (eds.) Viral Hepatitis: A Contemporay Assessment of Etiology, Epidemiology, Pathogenesis and Prevention, pp. 491–505 (Philadelphia: Franklin Institute Press)

7. Maupas, P., Goudeau, A., Coursaget, P., Drucker, J. and Bagros, P. (1978). Hepatitis B vaccine: efficacy in high-risk settings, a two year study. Intervirology, 10, 196

8. Hilleman, M.R., Bertland, A.U., Buynak, E.B., Lampson, G.P., McAleer, W.J., McLean, A.A., Roehm, R.R. and Tytell, A.A. (1978). Clinical and laboratory studies of HB_sAg vaccine. In: G.N. Vyas, S.N. Cohen and R. Schmid (eds.) Viral Hepatitis: A Contemporary Assessment of Etiology, Epidemiology, Pathogenesis and Prevention, pp. 525–537 (Philadelphia: Franklin Institute Press)

9. Szmuness, W. (1979). Large scale efficacy trials of hepatitis B vaccines in the USA: baseline data and protocols. J. Med. Virol., 4, 327

10. Skelly, J., Howard, C.R., and Zuckerman, A.J. (1979). Analysis of hepatitis B surface antigen components solubilised with Triton X-100. J. Gen. Virol., 44, 679

11. Mishiro, S., Imai, M., Takahashi, K., Machida, A., Gotanda, T., Miyakawa, Y. and Mayumi, M. (1980). A 49,000 dalton polypeptide bearing all antigenic determinants and full immunogenicity of 22nm hepatitis B surface antigen particles. J. Immunol., 124, 1589

12. Pederson, D.L., Roberts, I.M. and Vyas, G.N. (1977). Partial amino acid sequence of two major component polypeptides of hepatitis B

surface antigen. Proc. Natl. Acad. Sci. USA, 74, 1350

13. Simons, K., Helenius, A., Leonard, K., Sarvas, M. and Gething, M.J. (1978). Formation of protein micelles from amphiphillic membrane proteins. Proc. Natl. Acad. Sci. USA, 75, 5306

14. Skelly, J., Howard, C.R. and Zuckerman, A.J. (1980). Hepatitis B polypeptide vaccine preparation in micelle form. (Submitted for publication)

15. Gerety, R.J., Tabor, E., Purcell, R.H. and Tyeryar, F.J. (1979). Summary of an International Workshop on Hepatitis B vaccines. J. Inf. Dis., 140, 642

16. Schild, G. (1974). In: Influenza Vaccines – Summary of influenza workshop. J. Inf. Dis., 129, 766

17. Pasek, M., Goto, T., Cilbert, W., Zink, B., Scaller, H., Mackay, P., Leadbetter, G. and Murray, K. (1979). Hepatitis B virus genes and their expression in E. coli. Nature, 282, 575

18. Greenberg, H.B., Pollard, R.B., Lutwick, L.I., Gregory, P.B., Robinson, W.S. and Merigan, T.C. (1976). Effect of human leucocyte interferon on hepatitis B virus infection in patients with chronic active hepatitis. N. Engl. J. Med., 295, 517

19. Scullard, G.H., Alberti, A., Wansbrough-Jones, M.H., Howard, C.R., Eddleston, A.L.W.F., Zuckerman, A.J., Cantell, K. and Williams, R. (1979). Effects of leucocyte interferon on hepatitis B virus replication and immune responses in patients with chronic hepatitis B infection. J. Clin. Lab. Immunol., 1, 277

20. Merigan, T.C. and Robinson, W.S. (1978). Antiviral therapy in HBV infection. In: G.N. Vyas, S.B. Cohen and R. Schmid (eds.) Viral Hepatitis: A Contemporay Assessment of Etiology, Epidemiology, Pathogenesis and Prevention. pp. 575-579 (Philadelphia: Franklin Institute Press)

21. Desmyter, J., Ray, M.B., De Groote, J., Bradbourne, A.F., Desmet, V.J., Edy, V.G., Billiau, A., De Somer, P. and Mortelmans,

J. (1976). Administration of human fibroblast interferon in chronic hepatitis B infection. Lancet, 2, 645

22. Kingham, J.G.C., Ganguly, Z., Sharri, D., Mendelson, R., McGuire, M.J., Holgate, S.J., Cartwright, T., Scott, G.M., Richards, M.B. and Wright R. (1978). Treatment of HB$_s$Ag-positive chronic active hepatitis with human fibroblast interferon. Gut, 19, 91

23. Galvao, P.A.A. and Castro, I.O. (1974). Treatment of acute viral hepatitis with a new antiviral compound. Rev. Bras. Clin. Ter., 3, 221

24. Huggins, D. and Pereira, G.J.M. (1977) O emprego do virazole como dedida terapeutica da hepatite aguda por virus. Revta. Bras. Med., 34, 307

25. Denes, A.E., Ebert, J.W., Berquist, K.R., Murphy, B.L. and Maynard, J.E. (1976). Antiviral effects of Virazole in chronic hepatitis B surface antigen-seropositive chimpanzees. Antimicrob. Agents Chemother. 10, 571

26. Zuckerman, A.J., Thornton, A., Howard, C.R., Tsiquaye, K.N., Jones, D.M. and Brambell, M.R. (1978). Hepatitis B outbreak among chimpanzees at the London Zoo. Lancet, 2, 652

27. Pollard, R.B., Smith, J.L., Neal, E.A., Gregory, P.B., Merigan, T.C. and Robinson, W.S. (1978) Effect of Vidarabine on chronic hepatitis B virus infection. J. Am. Med. Assoc., 239, 1648

28. Chadwick, R.G., Bassendine, M.F., Cawford, E.M., Thomas, H.C. and Sherlock, S. (1978). HB$_s$Ag-positive chronic liver disease: inhibition of DNA polymerase activity by vidarabine. Br. Med. J., 2, 531

29. Sonnenfield, G., Mandel, A.D. and Merigan, T.C. (1977). The immunosuppressive effect of type II mouse interferon preparations on antibody production. Cell. Immunol., 34, 193

30. Trinchieri, G. and Santoli, D. (1979). Anti-viral activity induced by culturing lymphocytes with tumor-derived or virus-transformed cells.

J. Exp. Med., <u>147</u>, 1314

31. Zarling, J.M., Eskra, L., Borden, E.C., Horoszewicz, J. and Carter, W.A. (1979). Activation of human natural killer cells cytotoxic for human leukaemia cells by purified interferon. J. Immunol., <u>123</u>, 63

32. Minato, N., Bloom, B.R., Jones, C., Holland, J. and Reid, L.M. (1979). Mechanism of rejection of virus persistently infected tumor cells by athymic nude mice. J. Exp. Med., <u>149</u>, 1117

ACKNOWLEDGEMENTS

The programme of hepatitis B vaccine research at the London School of Hygiene and Tropical Medicine is generously supported by the Wellcome Trust, and in part by the Department of Health and Social Security and Organon BV, Oss, Holland.

I am indebted to my colleagues Professor Arie Zuckerman and Dr. J. Skelly for advice and helpful discussions.

Discussion

<u>Prof. Stewart:</u>   Am I to understand that this work is only done in chronic active hepatitis? Can it not be used effectively in the acute phase?

<u>Dr. Howard:</u>   I am not aware of any detailed controlled studies that have been done on acute hepatitis B. I do not know that there are very strong grounds for trying out these drugs in acute hepatitis patients.

<u>Prof. Stewart:</u>   It is supposed to have a relatively high mortality - which is what everyone got rather excited about.

Dr. Howard: There have been studies. I am not saying there have not. But there have been very few studies that have been well controlled.

Dr. Thomas: We have done some studies with our monophosphate, and as Dr. Howard pointed out, we have only found it to have an effect in the E-antigen positive DNA polymerase positive patients and this phase in acute hepatitis is over by the time of clinical presentation. I think Interferon has been tried in some acute hepatitis and fulminant hepatitis patients. But I think this was on a last ditch basis, in that these patients had already had evidence of clearance of the virus, they were E-antigen negative, and HBS titres were falling at the time when the therapy was instigated.

Prof. Stewart: What about in animals?

Dr. Howard: I do not think any of us have that many animals that we can actually try those particular drugs out in chimpanzees. All of our chimpanzees in our units were chronically infected before they came to us. In the light of the pressure to understand non-A, non-B, we have not felt that it is necessarily a priority to look at these particular agents in chimpanzees acutely infected with hepatitis.

Dr. Stewart: And they would not be expected to work – is that what you are saying? Everyone got excited about hepatitis B because this has an appreciable mortality in the acute stage, which varies between 5 and 50 per cent, and that is why it was considered important.

Dr. Howard: Yes. But I think that, as Dr. Thomas has already pointed out, the critical thing here with chronic active hepatitis is the ongoing virus replication and very high levels which can be identified with two particular markers associated with complete virus. And I do make that distinction. There are lots of virus-like particles. There are double shelled forms that are empty. In the normal acute case, and this has been shown very clearly, both in the early Willowbrook studies that have been looked at in retrospect and also in the chimpanzee studies, that the peak of virus replication occurs very often before the patient presents himself to the clinician, and that those markers — that allow the efficacy of these particular compounds to be comfortably assessed — are not there to do this particular type of study. If the patient has demonstrable levels of DNA polymerase and E antigen, then that may be so, but in the vast majority of cases it is very difficult to find those two markers, and it is those two markers that so far in treatment of chronic active hepatitis have played such a vital role in understanding the effect of these compounds on the virus replication.

General Discussion

Prof. Bloom: To come back to my earlier question, what should the people who are not associated with a specialised liver unit be doing when they are faced with a young man who has persistently abnormal liver function tests, a spleen tip palpable and an enlarged liver. Should we be doing a liver biopsy? Is there any value in it? Or is there any possible treatment available?

Prof. MacSween: If I can perhaps interpret what others might say. I think in such a situation, there are strong indications for investigating the patient on the basis of his having some suspected liver disease. The payoff, unfortunately, is that we do not as yet have any therapy that we can give these patients with any degree of certainty that it will either prevent further progression of the disease or cure liver disease which may still be at a relatively early 'acute' or 'sub-acute' phase.

Dr. Triger: If we ever find an effective or a potentially effective way of treating any of these diseases which we are still — as we have heard today — in the process of defining, we will not be able to assess the efficacy of treatment unless we have some idea about the rate of progression, and even if there is a disease that is progressing. For that reason, many of us feel that some objective assessment is important. For lack of a better way we really do have to look on biopsy as a useful tool at the moment.

Hopefully, we could use liver biopsy, and we may with that as a standard, be able to involve other techniques. One possibility is CT scanning, which might in the future be usable in that way. Perhaps pro-collagen, as Dr. Thomas mentioned, is another. But we have really got to come back to our standard, which at the moment is in Prof. Scheuer's field.

Prof. Bloom: What I am pressing to establish is whether this is regarded as a semi-investigative process which should be confined to those doing work on liver disease, or do the panellists think that in an ordinary haemophilia unit, without close contact with a specialised liver unit, we should be asking a physician who deals with these disorders to do a liver biopsy in a haemophiliac without any possible prospect of immediately effective treatment in the clinical situation.

Dr. Thomas: I would have thought, in direct answer to that last point, that liver biopsy is much safer if done by someone doing a lot, and therefore most would agree that it would be better to have the biopsy done by someone from a specialist unit. But I think that one goes back to the problem that Prof. MacSween has highlighted, that is that at the moment we have nothing of tangible benefit to offer them, so why define that they have progressive inflammatory liver lesions. The only way that we shall see an advance in terms of development of treatment is to have an equivalent of the sort of markers that Dr. Howard described, a DNA polymerase if indeed there is such an enzyme associated with a non-A, non-B hepatitis and then when those are available, we should have to start on the laborious process of testing out the same anti-viral agents as have been used, and are being used in hepatitis B. The first phase.must be the biological one where we try to look for methods of measuring viral replication, then to see perhaps in a non-haemophiliac population, what effect the anti-viral agents have, and then, with the knowledge of the natural history only accrued by biopsy in haemophiliac patients with the disease, we would be then in a position to bring to bear these biological tests and anti-viral therapies in this group of patients. I am afraid the timescale is many years.

Prof. Bloom: That has helped to answer the question. Dr. Thomas is saying that an odd histology report from a liver biopsy tucked away in the notes now is of little value unless it is done at a centre which is actively engaged in liver investigation.

Prof. Stewart: Yes, but it would be of value to him to document what happened to the patient and the no-treatment episode. That would be of value to them if they ever did get any way to assess it, because they will have the natural history of the untreated case.

Dr. Thomas: This is an unusual situation, where there is a national body co-ordinating the care of these patients, and it is an ideal circumstance within which to gain information, albeit in small parcels from the units and the physicians concerned, but together making up something that would be worthwhile in understanding the natural history of this condition. It might be argued that we should see what the natural history is in non-haemophiliac patients, but we then ultimately have the issue as to whether it behaves in the same way in the haemophiliacs who are getting the higher dosage more frequently.

Prof. Stewart: So the best thing we can do at the moment is document it?

Dr. Thomas: Yes, but in collaboration with the local hepatology unit.

Prof. Stewart: So support those involved in the research enormously, but meanwhile we document all the others and see what happens.

Anonymous: I wonder if I could also add, it seems to be as a result of today's discussions, that in the interim, and as a possibly prophylactic measure, that if one is looking after a child with haemophilia, then one should limit any concentrate one gives to British-produced concentrate.

Dr. Craske: I do not know that that will necessarily follow. I do not think we yet have enough evidence to say whether NHS concentrate has a lower incidence of symptomless hepatitis.

Prof. MacSween: This afternoon has been an interesting and exciting one, and I hope that collaboration between haematologists and hepatologists will provide an answer to the problems that have been discussed.

SECTION II   Therapy
for
Haemophilia

Opening remarks

A. L. Bloom

It is remarkable to reflect that until 20 years ago treatment for haemophilia was in the main restricted to blood transfusion and the infusion of fresh frozen plasma, and even this treatment was available only to a few patients; thus 11 were treated at my own centre in Cardiff in 1964. The provision of freeze-dried concentrates pioneered at Oxford, London and Stockholm and prepared from human and animal blood during the early 1960's represented a notable advance but supplies of the human material at that time were minute and its potency low. The solubility of the porcine and bovine Factor VIII preparations then available was poor and the thrombocytopenia, occasional reactions, and eventual resistance limited their therapeutic value.

The two developments which revolutionised haemophilia management were the discovery by Judith Pool and her colleagues, of cryoprecipitate in 1964 to 1965, and the provision of home therapy. In fact the latter really developed from the former because most of the present generation of intermediate and high purity concentrates start off as a cryoprecipitate of one form or other and are indispensable for an adequate home treatment programme.

Successful though this treatment has been many problems remain to be solved, notably the high incidence of abnormal liver function tests and various forms of hepatitis discussed in detail elsewhere in this symposium and also the development of inhibitor to Factor VIII. The immunological problems of haemophilia therapy feature in this session. Evidence concerning the efficiency of Factor IX-prothrombin concentrates, be they non-activated, fortuitously activated or purposefully contact-activated, has been controversial; thus the two papers in the present session are timely. The first of these records the results of a controlled clinical trial of one preparation and the second a rather more anecdotal account of the use of another. Useful though these preparations seem to be, they do not match the effectiveness of Factor VIII concentrate in responsive haemophiliacs and their cost is enormous so that the treatment of these resistant patients continues to pose many problems.

The hepatitis risk highlights the desirability of avoiding blood products in susceptible patients such as the mildly affected haemophiliac or those with von Willebrand's disease. The possibility of using deamino-D-arginine vasopressin (DDAVP) in conjunction with antifibrinolytic therapy for short courses of treatment in this type of patient therefore represents a notable advance.

For the future perhaps we may look forward to the preparation of less expensive and more highly purified preparations of procoagulant Factor VIII and of the von Willebrand factor using the polyelectrolyte method; possibly even porcine procoagulant Factor VIII separated by this method may find a new role in some patients with antibody. It remains to be seen if the oral administration of Factor VIII in lipid vesicles or liposomes – surely a dream of all haemophiliacs – will develop into a practical and effective method of treatment.

Fascinating though these scientific developments may be, therapeutic advances are of little value without effective delivery of health care which is acceptable to the patient, capable of being provided and within the budget of individuals or agencies. The usage of Factor VIII concentrates in the U.K. has been assessed accurately because of the organisation of Haemophilia Centre Directors and the returns effectively collated at the Oxford Centre; the current usage of 50 million units was forecast in 1975. The most recent data indicate that the annual requirement will rise to 85 million units by 1985 due perhaps to developments such as home treatment and limited prophylaxis. It is the experience of most haematologists that crude cryoprecipitate is not a suitable material for home treatment and the shortfall of Health Service produced freeze-dried intermediate or high purity concentrate in the U.K. is likely to reach 60 million units per annum by the middle of this decade. Are we to continue to purchase this from commercial sources at a cost of about £5 million per annum or entrust our fractionation facilities to the pressures of private enterprise, or would the money be better spent in providing and maintaining adequate plasma collection and fractionation facilities within the NHS? One may well prefer the latter option. Many of these problems are echoed around the world and it is appropriate therefore that this session commences with a discussion from the U.S.A. on the organisation, provision, cost and complications of a haemophilia home therapy programme.

7

The cost of care

L. M. Aledorf and M. Diaz

Haemophilia, a genetically inherited chronic disease, necessitates life-long health care. This chapter discusses in detail the current approach to haemophilia treatment. Early diagnosis and carrier detection has made possible the offer of intelligent options for family planning. Genetic counsellors, with psycho-social back-up are prepared to offer support for the emotional needs that the impact of this information may produce[1]. Major emphasis on patient and family education programmes have made those involved with the disease aware of optimal care programmes. The multi-discipline comprehensive care approach to these patients has served as an effective means for regular medical, dental, laboratory and psycho-social evaluation and on-going care[2].

This comprehensive care, team approach requires a large number of personnel gathered together in one place. These teams can effectively care for large numbers of patients over a large region. They can be itinerant, relate to distant primary care physicians, and develop satellite programmes. These teams are costly to maintain but are the core for a regionalised network of treatment programmes which can assure superior care for haemophiliacs. It is rare that such a team can be put together and maintained by an institution without outside financial support. Chapters of the National Haemophilia Foundation in some instances are helpful in either partial or full support of a single member of the team. In some state haemophilia programmes, financial support is given for either a core state laboratory or a member of the comprehensive team. In rare programmes third party reimbursement on a fee for service basis can help support a part of the team. Much of the physician time given to these programmes is voluntary.

*This paper was read by Dr. M. Hilgartner

At present, the most important form of support for comprehensive centres in the United States is from the Federal Government. In 1975, three million dollars was given for the development of a national network of comprehensive haemophilia diagnostic and treatment centres[3]. These are competed for, centrally reviewed and awarded via the Health Services Administration. Twenty-one centres are funded. In addition, other non-funded comprehensive centres exist[4]. The funds are used primarily for personnel which programmes could not support on their own. The centres have demonstrated in a short time that more patients are served, more services delivered and a large number of community agencies interact with these patients. Almost 30% of the nations haemophiliacs are served by these centres.

The unique feature of haemophilia, versus other chronic diseases, is the continued dependence of these patients on blood products. In a recent study the average demand for blood products for a large number of haemophiliacs throughout the United States, was about 40,000 units of factor VIII per patient per year. It is clear from this evaluation that more factor is used by the more severely involved patient, and that home care patients infuse more often and use more product[5]. Severe home care patients use almost 60,000 Factor VIII units per year. These figures were corroborated by prior sampling of non-study centres[6].

Current treatment of haemophilia has moved the haemophiliac from an in-hospital patient to a more independent ambulatory person capable of receiving diagnostic and therapeutic programmes in an out-patient facility, or at home or work. "Self therapy" frequently called home care, has substantially altered the lifestyle and productivity of these patients.

In the United States the place of treatment, and type of product used is frequently determined by the ability to pay. In a pluralistic society such as that found in the United States health care systems vary from region to region, and are frequently different even within a given state. A major consideration for every programme for its individual patient is - what is the impact of any given treatment regimen on "out-of-pocket" expense, and can the patient or his family afford it?

The choice of product is frequently a matter of cost. In many centres where a blood bank has a major vested interest in haemophilia, cryoprecipitate is produced cheaply and used extensively. In general, however, cryoprecipitate is not inexpensive and its quality is variable. Concentrates vary in price. The price varies little from product to product, but a given product may be priced very differently in various parts of the country at the same time. This is frequently due to (a) long term contracts, (b) volume and (c) bids.

Table 1   Extent Of Haemophilia Treatment Centre Coverage In The United States

States and parts of states without federal funding for haemophilia treatment centres	States with State funding for haemophilia treatment (blood products and/or treatment programmes)	States and territories without federal funding and state funding for haemophilia treatment
Alabama	Alabama	Kansas
Arkansas (Almost entire state except N.E. corner)	California	Maryland
	Colorado	Nebraska
Florida (Southern)	Georgia	Nevada
Georgia (North West)	Illinois	North Dakota
Illinois (Entire state except N.W. corner)	Indiana	Oklahoma
	Kentucky	Puerto Rico
Kansas	Louisiana	Virgin Islands
Kentucky	Minnesota	
Louisiana	Mississippi	
Maine (Northern)	Missouri	
Maryland	New Hampshire	
Mississippi (Entire state except North)	New Jersey	
	Ohio	
Missouri	Oregon	
Nebraska	Pennsylvania	
Nevada	Rhode Island	
New York (North Eastern)	South Carolina	
North Dakota	Tennessee	
Ohio	Texas	
Oklahoma	Virginia	
Pennsylvania (Western)	Wisconsin	
Tennessee (Entire state except West)		

Texas (Central & Northern)
Washington (Entire state
except South)
West Virginia (Entire state
except Southern tip)

Sources: (1) State & Federal Resources Guide For Hemophiliacs, 1979,
              published by the National Hemophilia Foundation.
          (2) FY-1980 Federally Funded Comprehensive Hemophilia
              Treatment Centers List.
          (3) Map produced by Health Services Administration, DHEW,
              February 28, 1980.

Table 1. Kindly provided by Mrs. Deidre Richardson, Acting Executive
          Director, National Haemophilia Foundation.

State funded haemophilia programmes, (Table 1) in the main, support the cost of product. Some also underwrite parts of the care system (i.e. diagnostic X-ray). State legislation is variable, administered in different state agencies. Sometimes closely aligned to National Hemophilia Foundation chapters (i.e. Oregon) and occasionally part of broader based entities, such as Crippled Childrens' programmes or Genetic Disease or Handicapped Persons programmes (i.e. California). In general, however, the support for concentrate has an upper limit, beginning after all other sources are used (private insurance) and all registered families are eligible at all ages without regard for income level. Many states reimburse for product used at patient or doctor discretion. Other programmes purchase all product at open bid and then distribute. Thus price of final product can strongly influence what is used. These state programmes have been critical for elevating the level of care made available to involved patients. In addition they have provided patient identification, and the collection of valuable data on product utilisation, health care status and laboratory assessment.

Many other countries have dealt with health care by instituting some form of national health insurance. Our nation does not have a uniform system for insuring health care delivery. The poor can avail themselves of Medicaid, SSI, and Crippled Childrens' programmes. The latter usually only covers patients under 21. Even these programmes differ regionally in terms of what they cover. As factor replacement is most often the major part of the cost of care, its reimbursement is the key part of underwriting care. In almost all of the aforementioned reimbursement programmes, factor is reimbursed for in-patient emergency room use. The underwriting of factor for out-of-hospital care (home care) however, remains variable. When not covered, patients are usually not able to take part in this type of self care. It has been previously shown that as out-of-pocket expenses increase, patients and their families are less likely to follow prescribed treatment programmes[7]. Private insurance programmes may vary as much as state and city funded health care programmes. Blue Cross and Blue Shield programmes within the same region may be widely divergent. One consistent problem that patients faced was that out-of-hospital blood products that are utilised are often not covered by third party payers. This is also true of many private insurance programmes.

This variability of insurance has made treatment centres become very aware of the need for evaluating the finacial resources of each patient and his family. A treatment programme cannot be realistically prescribed without such an evaluation. Recent publications[8,9] outline the key elements for financial assessment as well as counselling. This kind of financial evaluation was the major impetus for the treaters through local chapters of the National Hemophilia Foundation and the National Hemophilia office, to begin campaigns to alter policies of third party payers. These appeals have been met with success in many parts of this country. At present a large number of insurance carriers have altered their policies and home treatment programmes have begun to be underwritten and flourish. In addition, many union contracts now follow the lead of AT&T to cover home care treatment for patients with haemophilia. This coupled with state programmes which augment reimbursement, has made home therapy a major modality of treatment.

Programmes making decisions on therapy should carry out financial assessment on their patients and be aware of the financial impact of home care before prescribing it.

Table 2 demonstrates costs of total care when analysed for four patients before and after they were on a home care programme. These data were collected during the mid 1970's. The next Table (3) analyses three patients who were on home care programmes in 1975 which were reimbursed by third party payers[10]. In 1978 they reached 65 years of age and were now covered by Medicare which does not cover out-of-hospital transfusions. Of note in each case was a substantial increase in annual costs when not on home care. Of particular importance in the latter table is that despite the fact that these patients used more product in 1978 in comparison to 1975, the major cost differential was for in-patient days needed for transfusing the patient for bleeding episodes. These findings are consistent throughout the country. They clearly show the fiscal benefits of home care programmes and the needs for Medicare reform.

Table 2

Begun on home prescriptions	Annual cost before home prescriptions	Annual cost on home prescriptions
1. E.G. ...... November 1970	$ 9,437	$ 8,750
2. A.P. ...... February 1975	$13,765	$ 5,701
3. A.Y. ...... November 1974	$ 5,376	$ 6,377
4. S.A. ...... October 1974	$11,376	$ 6,074
Total	$39,954	$26,902

Table 2. Aledort LM: Amendments to the Medicare Programme. Hearings before the Subcommittee on Health, Committee on Ways and Means, House of Representatives, Ninety-Sixth Congress, First Session, 1979, pp. 200-204.

The pluralistic reimbursement programmes throughout the United States therefore are very important in determining the total cost of care, as well as the type of treatment programme used. The future tasks for us that remain are clear. We must continue to encourage proliferation of treatment centres and renewal of federal funds to support them in order to provide comprehensive care to all such patients. States which do not have special programmes for haemophilia must be provided with data as to why haemophilia care is cost effective and thus why states should help to underwrite such programmes.

Insurance carriers, Medicaid and Medicare programmes must be provided with clear cut evidence that out-of-hospital transfusions must be reimbursed, so that haemophiliacs can lead productive lives. Important additional information is that haemophilia is not the only disease which reimbursement for ambulatory transfusions would be cost effective. Red cells for sickle cell anaemia, thalassaemia and platelets for patients on chemotherapy can be administered on an ambulatory basis with significant savings if this procedure does not necessitate hospitalisation. Health care planners, involved in national health insurance must be made aware of the needs of our patients requiring chronic replacement therapy. When costs of therapy are met and a network of comprehensive care centres are assured continued existence, haemophiliacs can begin to believe that a near normal existence is possible.

Table 3

		Home care coverage 1975	Medicare No home care coverage 1978
		$	$
1	OPD	261	365
	Factor VIII	1,980	3,000
	In patient	0	3,216
		2,241	6,571
2	OPD	567	678
	Factor VIII	5,500	6,800
	In patient	0	3,680
		6,067	10,758
3	OPD	362	477
	Factor VIII	3,672	4,800
	In patient	0	3,800
		4,034	9,077

Table 3. Aledort LM: Amendments to the Medicare Programme. Hearings before the Subcommittee on Health, Committee on Ways and Means, House of Representatives, Ninety-Sixth Congress, First Session, 1979, pp. 200-204.

REFERENCES

1. Aledort, L.M. and working group (1977). Methods for the detection of haemophilia carriers: A memorandum. Bull. WHO, 55, 675

2. Gilbert, M. and Aledort, L.M. (1977). Comprehensive care in haemophilia: A team approach. Mt. Sinai. J. Med. 44, 313

3. Public Law 94-63, section 1131. Establishment of Hemophilia Diagnostic and Treatment Centres.

4. Directory of Haemophilia Treatment Centres. The National Hemophilia Foundation, 1979, pp 1-62

5. Aledort, L.M., Goodnight, S., Schwarz, J., Rao, V.J. and Shapiro, S. and inhibitor study group. NHLBI supported. Personal Communication.

6. Personal Communication. Aledort, L.M., Hilgartner, M., Levine, P., Linney, D., Eyster, E., Counts, R.

7. Levine, P. (1974). Efficacy of self therapy in haemophilia: A study of 72 patients with hemophilia A & B. N. Engl. J. Med., 291, 1381

8. Financial Counselling in Haemophilia. Prepared by David Linney, Financial Aids Officer, Great Lakes Hemophilia Foundation, Milwaukee Wisconsin, 1979, pp 1-9.

9. Financial Counselling Supplement. Prepared by David Linney, Financial Aids Officer, Great Lakes Hemophilia Foundation, Milwaukee Wisconsin, 1979, pp 1-13

10. Aledort L.M. (1979). Amendments to the Medicare Programme. Hearings before the Subcommittee on Health, Committee on Ways and Means, House of Representatives, Ninety-Sixth Congress, First Session, 1979, pp 200-204

Discussion

Prof. Bloom   As far as we are concened in the UK it raises a lot of questions. Dr. Hilgartner mentioned that the average use is 40,000–44,000 units per year, and yet when you started the talk you emphasised the difficulties in funding the treatment. Does that 40,000–44,000 represent an average over the whole spectrum of haemophiliacs, those who cannot afford treatment or who do not get it because of that reason, or is it an average taking into account all the patients with haemophilia?

Dr. Hilgartner: The 40,000 units from the State of Pennsylvania takes in everyone. In the State of Pennsylvania they do support product costs. Unfortunately our figures are spotty because the way that the product is paid for varies per state. The 44,000 units figure from the Inhibitor Study Group again came from centres in which care is supported. In most of our areas, the patient can receive care, but care unfortunately has to be in hospital. We have had the greatest difficulty in getting care on a home care basis, a home infusion basis, and that is where the majority of the problems exist. Patients can get care in hospital, and we still do have areas in which that is the primary way in which care is given, but they are becoming less and less. We assume now that we have between 40 and 50 per cent of the known haemophiliacs in the country on home care, so that in the whole ability to pay – the system is improving but it is a very long and very tedious one to get it for all the patients.

Prof. Bloom: I am sure that it will not have escaped Directors of Haemophilia Centres here that if we extrapolate the figures that Prof. Hilgartner has just given us to our own situation, we could anticipate usage in the UK going up to at least 80 million units a year straight away. This is worth bearing in mind. We are currently running at about 45 million units.

Dr. Crawford: May I take the argument further and say that I have just worked out that 40 kilounits per patient per annum amounts to 2.4

million units per million population, provided that we are treating about 60 haemophiliacs per million population. I wondered if the figures did refer to all haemophiliacs, or just to all haemophiliacs who had a bleeding episode in the year reported.

Dr. Hilgartner: It refers to the patients who have had a bleeding episode in that particular year. We do not have, as yet, a good system for cataloguing all the patients in the country. We are just in the process of developing that, so that our numbers still may be suspect.

Dr. Crawford: In any given year do you expect to see about two-thirds or four-fifiths of haemophiliacs?

Dr. Hilgartner: Probably about two thirds.

Prof. Stewart: What is the function of the genetic counsellor? Its an X-linked disease. What does he do?

Dr. Hilgartner: Prof. Graham will be going into this in detail. The genetic counsellor not only talks to the new families who appear, and discusses what the reproductive choices may be, and finds whether there is/there is not a carrier in the family, but the counsellor is available for all of the haemophiliacs themselves, and it is surprising to recognise how few of the patients know that all of their daughters are likely to be carriers. Very few patients seem to recognise that fact, or even to take it into consideration in planning their own families. The genetic counsellor is available to both the males and the females, and is particularly available to the siblings. The siblings require a great deal of help, not only psychologically, in facing the fact that they are possibly carriers, but in planning their families.

Prof. Abilgaard: Many of us serve as our own genetic counsellors. Very few centres have a specific genetic counsellor to do the job that many of us do ourselves.

Dr. Kernoff: Assuming that the figure of 44,000 units does represent what goes on in the USA it is obviously more than we are using here. Is that because we are under-treating patients, or is it because you are over-treating patients in the USA?   We are in the position of having to make targets - as was discussed in yesterday's session - and we should like to know if it is realistic to make a target based on what happens in the USA?

Dr. Hilgartner: We do not quite know ourselves whether we are over-treating.   There was a great variation between the Centres themselves, whose figures were brought into this.   There were two or three Centres which seemed to use a figure that was 10,000 units higher per year, and there were other Centres that were down as low as 20,000.   The only way we shall be able to say who is right is to see in ten years what the joint situation is for the patients in each of those Centres.   It is a long-term process, and we do not yet know.   There are several Centres which were much impressed with Dr. Preston's article in the Lancet in which he showed that they are certainly using a much, much lower figure in the U.K. than we had been using.   And there are various groups which are now trying to duplicate that particular use, going down to as low as 7 to 10 units for the treatment of joints.   Only in the long term shall we be able to answer that question.   We do not think prophylaxis is necessary for every patient, but whether we are still using too much for the treatment of ordinary joint bleeding is a question we cannot yet answer: it will take another five years.

Prof. Stewart: I understood Dr. Hilgartner's figure to refer only to patients who had been treated that year.   Is it not true that our figures take the total amount and divide it by the total number of haemophiliacs, which is not the same, because not everyone gets treated every year?

Prof. Bloom: That is not true.   It is the usage per patient treated during any one year.

Dr. Jones: I would like to add a rider to Dr. Kernoff's question. There is one variable that we can get out today without waiting for five or six years, and that is the number of bleeds that stop with one treatment. Could Dr. Hilgartner tell us the proportion of your own patients who report that their bleeds stop with one treatment at the sort of dosage regime that produces 44,000 units a year.

Dr. Hilgartner: I do not know that we really can get that answer, because we would have to get out of our data how many patients have a chronic joint. There are many chronic joints that do not stop with only one treatment. I would guess that a third of our patients take a second treatment.

Dr. Jones: Do they have a second treatment because they know that if they do not they will continue to bleed, or do they take it as a prophylactic shot?

Dr. Hilgartner: There are maybe half a dozen who take it prophylactically, and the others do it because the episode has not resolved.

Dr. Aronstam: Dr. Hilgartner's dose for propylaxis is about three times the size of the dose I would normally use. We find between a 60 or 70 per cent reduction in bleeding frequency on our dose. Could Dr. Hilgartner quote a figure for the reduction in bleeding frequency on prophylaxis on your dose?

Dr. Hilgartner: The patients who are on prophylaxis may break through with a bleeding episode once or twice a year, and that is all.

Prof. Bloom: It is interesting that in the US, where there is close financial control, and doctors therefore have some idea of the overall cost of hospital treatment, which it is perhaps very difficult for physicians in the UK to get hold of, when the patients are put on home treatment the financial adviser finds that the cost of treatment is reduced. I do not know if that is a function of the dosages used, but it is something that is not taken into account sufficiently in the UK by the administrators.

Dr. Hilgartner: If anything, the amount of product increases for the first year or so the patients are on therapy. The cost reduction is due entirely to the decrease in physician fee and outpatient emergency room fee.

Prof. Bloom: Fees still come into the fact that we have got to get paid one way or another, so it is still relevant.

8

The effect of activated prothrombin-complex concentrate (FEIBA) on joint and muscle bleedings in patients with haemophilia A with an inhibitor to Factor VIII

J. L. van Geijlswijk

A double blind study was carried out on 15 haemophilia A patients with inhibitors using FEIBA (Immuno) as the investigational drug and prothrombin complex (Prothromplex, Immuno) as the alternate therapy.

It was the object of the study to evaluate the efficacy of the two preparations in the control of joint, muscle and open haemorrhages. The comparison was based on single doses of FEIBA (100 U/kg) against single doses of Prothromplex (60 U/kg). For each patient a stratification was made indentifying potential bleeding locations in joints and muscles; right knee, left knee, right elbow, left elbow etc. A list of randomised pairs for Prothromplex and FEIBA was drawn up for each joint before the study. With each pair of treated episodes, both the patient and attending physician had to decide by a list of various parameters which of the two therapies was more effective. In addition, the result of each treatment was evaluated by a four degree scale, the evaluations ranging from excellent, moderate, nil to deterioration.

The selection criteria the patients had to meet in order to participate in the trial were the following; the inhibitor titre should at least once have been higher than five Bethesda units, the patient should be a high responder, more than one bleeding per month in the preceding year, no signs of liver failure, willing to co-operate and to stay in hospital during 24 hours at least.

With regard to the use of Prothromplex it must be emphasised that a purely neutral placebo could not be used, but a material with its own beneficial effect. In itself, this was not a problem, on the contrary, the opportunity was taken to measure the effect of the action of a prothrombin-complex concentrate.

Treatment was started as soon as possible after the start of bleeding and the administration was as fast as feasible. A second treatment was allowed for muscle bleedings after 12 hours and for open bleedings after 6 hours. Other treatment, for instance bed-rest, bandages, analgesics and so on, was optional with the exception of anti-fibrinolytic drugs, which were avoided because of the risk of disseminated intra-vascular coagulation.

Evaluation took place prior to treatment and 1 hour, 6 hours and 24 hours after treatment. The criteria used were; severity of pain and rate of improvement, the circumference of joint or muscle, the limitations of movement, the subjective reaction of the patient answering the question, "do you feel better, the same or worse?", the quantity of analgesics required, and at the 24 hour evaluation the patient, as well as the investigator, had to report whether they thought that the treatment had been effective, partially effective, doubtful or not effective. Moreover, they had to compare the result with the result of a previous treatment for the same location. Other evaluation criteria were, the time required for complete convalescence and the absence from school or work.

In order to standardise the technique of measurement, the doctors took part in three pre-trial evaluations and, if possible, the same investigator performed all measurements of a single episode.

Laboratory Data

The assay of haemoglobin and haematocrit was used to detect significant blood loss particularly in muscle bleedings. The assays of platelets, fibrin degradation products, fibrino-peptide A and the ethanol gelation test were done to detect any intravascular coagulation. The liver function tests were done every 2 months or more if necessary. A rise in the inhibitor level could indicate the presence of Factor VIII in the material administered. Assays of antithrombin III and Factor V were also performed.

Results

The total number of haemorrhages treated in the course of the study included 117 joint bleedings, 29 muscle bleedings and 4 open bleedings. Since the number of open bleedings was so small only joint and muscle bleedings were used for the statistical evaluation after Wilcoxon/ Mann-Witney.

Summary of data: number of patients   15
                  number of incidents   150
                  joint   117
                  muscle   29
                  open   4
                  analysable in pairs   51
                  joint   40
                  muscle   11

Most of the joint bleeding occurred in the knee, the elbow and the ankle, as many on the right as on the left side. At the end of each single treatment the patient and the investigator had to judge whether the given drug had been effective or not. The results are below:

Total effect according to the patient:

	FEIBA		Prothromplex	
Effective	26	(41,2%)	14	(25,0%)
Partially effective	16	(25,3%)	12	(21,4%)
Dubious	4	(6,3%)	9	(16,0%)
Without any effect	17	(26,9%)	21	(37,5%)
	63		56	

p = 0.414 (Wilcoxon/Mann-Witney)

Total effect according to the investigator:

	FEIBA		Prothromplex	
Effective	32	(41,5%)	19	(26,3%)
Partially effective	18	(23,3%)	19	(26,3%)
Dubious	10	(12,9%)	14	(19,4%)
Without any effect	17	(22,0%)	20	(27,7%)
	77		72	

p = 0.0749

The number of cases judged by the investigator is greater because there were a number of children involved and they could not do their own reporting.

There is a difference in the total numbers of bleedings treated by FEIBA and Prothromplex because not all pairs have been completed and by chance FEIBA has been given more frequently than the placebo.

The high percentages for the effectiveness of the Prothromplex proves that it has its own beneficial effect as already mentioned.

Below, the results of the comparison in pairs from the point of view of the patient and the investigator respectively:

Comparison In Pairs

	According to patient		According to investigator	
	FEIBA	Prothromplex	FEIBA	Prothromplex
Better	9	3	13	6
Dubious	1	1	4	5
Same	1	3	4	11
Worse	2	5	2	6
	13	12	23	28

p = 0.0327   p = 0.0084

In the first column are the results when FEIBA was given for the second episode and compared by the patient and investigator respectively with the alternate, given the first time for the same location. In the second column are the results of the comparison between Prothromplex and FEIBA when placebo-treatment followed the FEIBA-treatment.

In nine cases FEIBA was judged to be better when it was given second, but only in three cases did the patient find Prothromplex more effective, when it followed FEIBA treatment.

The measurement of joint mobility revealed a significant improvement of $p = 0.04$ after 6 hours and $p = 0.006$ after 24 hours.

The cephalin clotting time was considerably shortened ($p = 0.016$) with FEIBA in comparison to Prothromplex, however this also considerably shortened the cephalin clotting time as against the values before treatment. It must be said that no clear correlation could be found between the clinical improvement and shortening of the cephalin clotting time.

The inhibitor titre rose in two patients, remained the same in one, and decreased in twelve patients.

Three cases of hepatitis were reported, allergic-anaphylactoid reactions did not occur. There were no clinical or laboratory indications of disseminated intravascular coagulation or thromo-embolic processes.

SUMMARY

The double blind study outlined above, comparing single doses of FEIBA (100 U/kg) against Prothromplex (60 U/kg) revealed a significant benefit of FEIBA in the treatment of patients with haemophilia A with an inhibitor.

Discussion

Prof. Bloom: Dr. Geijlswijk has described a very carefully conducted clinical trial which I know was only made possible by the determination of the staff. All measurements were done by the same three individuals who got up in the middle of the night to measure joint movements frequently. It was a very carefully performed study.

Prof. Stewart: What was the time taken to go back to work?

Dr. Geijlswijk: Patients were advised to start work as soon as they were free of pain and the joints were able to move normally.

Prof. Stewart: And what was the difference between the FEIBA and the other treatment?

Dr. Geijlswijk: We thought that with the placebo the time off from work was shorter than with FEIBA.

Dr. Chediak: It seems that the placebo will produce a mean PTT of 34 seconds. Is that placebo indeed a placebo?

Dr. Geijlswijk: I have already explained that we realised it was not a real placebo. As I have already mentioned, our placebo has been investigated as a non-activated prothrombin complex against a real placebo.

Dr. Preston: Was the same batch of FEIBA used throughout the trial, and was the same batch of placebo used throughout the trial?

Dr. Geijlswijk: No. We used several batches.

Dr. Preston: I asked the question because some concern has been expressed in the past about interbatch variation in efficacy, certainly with FEIBA. That is certainly our experience and there are considerable differences.

Dr. Geijlswijk: Yes, it is true. Maybe later on we can try to find the differences between the batches that were used. But we have not calculated it up till now.

Dr. Rizza: Dr. Geijlswijk mentioned in an early slide that patients who were suffering from severe haemorrhage were not entered into the trial. Were they ever given Factor VIII?

Dr. Geijlswijk: No. We managed with FEIBA and blood transfusions. We did not use high dosages of Factor VIII.

Prof. Bloom: Was FEIBA used for the severe bleeds that were not reported in the trial?

Dr. Geijlswijk: Yes. We tried to start with FEIBA, and so far we have succeeded in stopping all the bleedings: the four bleedings mentioned here, and two severe bleedings into the abdominal wall with great blood loss.

Dr. Aronstam: I appreciate that patients were paired for bleeds at the same site. Was any allowance made for differences in the severity of the bleeds?

Dr. Geijlswijk: Yes. Later we did certain calculations and we saw that the effects of the FEIBA were strongest in the middle grade bleeders. The very severe bleedings and the slight bleedings did not react as well as the middle grade of bleeds.

Dr. Aronstam: Did the pairs actually compare bleeds of the same severity?

Dr. Geijlswijk: No. All bleeds were taken together.

Dr. Mayne: From experience within the trial and beyond the trial, has Dr. Geijlswijk found any of his inhibitor patients to always respond to FEIBA. I have about fourteen such patients, and of the fourteen two always respond very well to FEIBA and the others do not. Did Dr. Geijlswijk have any patients like that?

Prof. Bloom: Perhaps it could be put the opposite way. Were there any patients who did not respond to FEIBA?

Dr. Geijlswijk: We had the same experience. There were patients who always showed a good reaction, and there were patients who many times had a negative reaction. We had the same experience.

Dr. McClure: Dr. Geijlswijk mentioned that as a patient criterion, to determine if there were high responders, you gave them Factor VIII prior to the study. What was the dose of the Factor VIII and how much time was there between that dose and the one in the study?

Dr. Geijlswijk: We gave a dose to reach an expected level of 20 per cent, and we re-evaluated the levels at intervals of 14 days.

Prof. Bloom: Returning to the question of the number of batches of FEIBA, am I right in assuming that there were several batches of FEIBA, because in previous discussions I have had, I had been given to understand that only one batch of FEIBA was used.

Dr. Geijlswijk: I thought we had two batches.

Prof. Bloom: If people are interested in this, it would need to be cleared up a little. It is an important point.

9

Therapeutic use of DDAVP in haemophilia and von Willebrand's disease

C. A. Ludlam

The plasma Factor VIII concentration rises in reponse to a wide variety of physiological stimuli, e.g. exercise, pregnancy, and in many pathological conditions. Factor VIII levels can be increased pharmacologically by stimulation of $beta_2$-receptors[1,2] and by vasopressin and some of its synthetic analogues. Infusion of vasopressin intravenously, however, is also accompanied by contraction of smooth muscle in blood vessel walls, gastrointestinal tract and uterus and use of this property is made in the treatment of major gastrointestinal bleeding, particularly from oesophageal varices. It is possible that the analogue triglycyl-vasopressin may supersede the native molecule as a more useful therapeutic agent in this context and also for the treatment of menorrhagia[3]. The addition of the triglycyl residues delays the metabolism by the enzyme aminopeptidase[4]. Catabolism of infused vasopressin by this enzyme can also be reduced by removal of the N-terminal aminogroup. Substitution of D-arginine in position 8 for the naturally occurring L isomer not only inhibits metabolism by a carboxypeptidase but it also deprives the peptide of its smooth muscle stimulating property. When vasopressin is changed by these two latter modifications, the analogue desamino 8-D-arginine vasopressin (DDAVP) is produced. Although this has no vasopressor activity it retains the potent antidiuretic, Factor VIII and plasminogen activator stimulatory activity of the native molecule. It is the ability of DDAVP to increase plasma factor VIII levels that has ensured it an important place in the treatment of patients with mild haemophilia and von Willebrand's disease.

By using a variety of different vasopressin analogues the essential molecular features for its Factor VIII and plasminogen activator stimulating activity have been defined. The molecule must have a cyclic structure (dependent on the disulphide bond, although this can be replaced by a mono or dicarbo derivative), an aromatic residue in position 3 and a basic amino acid in position 8 with an omega aminogroup[5,6]. The mechanism by which the plasma concentration of these haemostatic components is raised is unknown. Both Factor VIIIRAG and probably plasminogen activator are synthesised by endothelial cells and all the evidence is consistent with the hypothesis that the DDAVP releases presynthesised molecules from such a store. There is no evidence that DDAVP interacts directly upon the endothelial cells, unlike adrenaline[5] and it seem probable that it releases one or more secondary chemical messengers, from an, at present unknown site, which in turn act upon endothelial cells. All the available evidence demonstrates that the Factor VIII that is liberated is identical to that which circulates under basal conditions[6,7].

DDAVP can be administered either intravenously or as snuff. As only relatively small doses are needed in diabetes insipidus it is given as snuff to patients with this disorder. Recently a "supersnuff", which contains a concentration of DDAVP ten times that of the ordinary snuff, has been produced and following nasal installation plasma Factor VIII levels increase. More research is needed on the value of this route of administration. In most studies in normal subjects and patients with Factor VIII deficiency states intravenous DDAVP has been used and this, at present, is the preferred route[8-10].

Intravenous infusion of DDAVP to normal subjects is followed by a brisk rise in all Factor VIII activities, i.e. Factor VIIIC, VIIICAG, VIIIRAG, and VIIIRISTOCOF, and plasminogen activator which reach a maximum at 30 minutes[6,7,10,11].

The response is dose related and reaches a maximum at 0.3 µg/kg and at this dose Factor VIII activities increase up to four-fold basal levels[12]. In mild haemophiliacs DDAVP also increases the Factor VIII concentration by up to four times the basal level[9,10], and the increase in VIIIRAG and VIIIRISTOCOF is much more prolonged than that of the VIIIC and VIIIRAG. In patients with basal Factor VIII levels of approximately 0.10 U/ml this can be increased to 0.4-0.5 U/ml for several hours whilst minor surgical procedures are accomplished. Although the anticipated response is observed in most haemophiliacs, occasional patients have been reported in whom the expected rise in all modalities was not observed. In two brothers with clinically severe haemophilia with basal Factor VIIIC levels at 0.05 U/ml, but undetectable VIIICAG, DDAVP resulted in an increase in all modalities of VIII except VIIICAG. It seems likely that these two patients have a functionally defective VIII and even although DDAVP increased the VIIIC level it is likely that this is not haemostatically competent[10].

In von Willebrand's disease (vWD) the response to vasopressin and its analogues is variable and depends upon the type of vWD. In patients with severe homozygous vWD, with grossly reduced Factor VIII activities (Type I)[13], DDAVP does not increase any of the Factor VIII activities or plasminogen activator; it is therefore not therapeutically useful in this uncommon form of vWD. In most patients with intermediate vWD and prolonged bleeding time (Type II) DDAVP increases all modalities of Factor VIII. Although in the original study by Mannucci[14] no shortening of the bleeding time was observed, in several other studies the rise in VIIIRISTOCOF was accompanied by a reduction in the bleeding time[10,15]. It appears that only a modest amount of VIIIRISTOCOF activity is needed (approximately 0.10 U/ml) to significantly shorten the bleeding time. One patient with type II vWD has been observed in whom DDAVP increased only the VIIIC and VIIICAG levels there being no concomitant rise in VIIIRAG, VIIIRISTOCOF or plasminogen activator. Furthermore neither adrenaline infusion or venous occlusion resulted in any significant increase in these latter activities[10]. Thus it appears that in some individuals with vWD the probable endothelial cell defect is more extensive than merely an inability of these cells to manufacture and release Factor VIIIRAG. In patients with vWD with normal bleeding time (type IV) DDAVP infusion is accompanied by a brisk response in all modalities of Factor VIII and plasminogen activator. Thus in most patients with vWD, provided each of the modalities of Factor VIII is detectable in the resting state, DDAVP appears to be a therapeutically useful way of temporarily improving haemostasis.

In mild haemophiliacs with basal Factor VIIIC of 0.10 U/ml and patients with vWD with basal VIIIRISTOCOF greater than 0.05 U/ml, DDAVP can be used to cover minor surgical procedures, e.g. dental extraction, lymph node biopsy, and tonsillectomy. It may have a place in the control of menorrhagia in vWD especially if this could be administered as supersnuff by the patient, but further studies are needed to ascertain this. When using DDAVP therapeutically in patients with Factor VIII deficiency states it is important to remember that it had other important effects besides raising the plasma concentration of Factor VIII. The enhanced fibrinolytic activity must be inhibited by prior administration of tranexamic acid (10 mg/kg intravenously). Some patients develop facial flushing and a slight tachycardia. These settle quickly if the injection is stopped for 1-2 minutes and continued at a lower rate. The antidiurectic activity lasts 24 hours and patients can suffer from cerebral oedma if the plasma osmolality falls significantly[16] but if patients are told to drink only a little then this is not a significant problem. One of the major drawbacks of DDAVP is that each successive injection is accompanied by a diminishing Factor VIII response. This tachyphylaxis is presumably due to exhaustion of the Factor VIII stores from which it is liberated and limits its usefulness for covering major surgery[8,17]. DDAVP is therefore the treatment of choice in mild haemophiliacs and most patients with vWD prior to minor surgery or to control external bleeding, e.g. epistaxis. It is easier to prepare than cryoprecipitate, but its major advantage is that it prevents this group of patients being exposed to blood products as they have a high chance of developing clinical hepatitis particularly following Factor VIII concentrates.

REFERENCES

1.   Gader, A.M.A., Clarkson, A.R. and Cash, J.D. (1973). The plasminogen activator and coagulation factor VIII response to adrenaline, noradrenaline, isoprenaline and salbutamol in man. Thrombosis Res., 2, 9

2.   Ingram, G.I.C., Jones, V.R., Hershgold, E.J., Densons, K.W.E. and Perkins, J.R. (1977). Factor VIII activity and antigen, platelet count and biochemical changes after adrenoceptor stimulation. Br. J. Haematol. 35, 81

3.   Pavlin, V., Flynn, M.J., Mulder, J.L. and Cort, J.H. (1978). The treatment of uterine bleeding with vasopressin hormonogen (Glypressin) − A pilot study. Br. J. Obstet. Gynaecol., 85, 11

4.   Cort, J.H. and Schwartz, I.L. (1978). An early look at the therapeutic uses of some new vasopressin analogs in gastroenterology. Yale J. Biol. Med., 51, 605

5.   Cash, J.D., Gader, A.M.A., Mulder, J.L. and Cort, J.H. (1978). Structure activity relations of the fibrinolytic response to vasopressins in man. Clin. Molec. Med., 54, 403

6.   Prowse, C.V., Sas, G., Gader, A.M.A., Cort, J.H. and Cash, J.D. (1979). Specificity in the factor VIII response to vasopressin infusion in man. Br. J. Haematol., 41, 437

7. Nilsson, I.M., Mikaelsson, M., Vilhart, H. and Walter, H. (1980). DDAVP factor VIII concentrate and its properties in vivo and in vitro. Thrombosis Res., 15, 263

8. Mannucci, P.M. Pareti, F.I., Ruggeri, Z.M. and Capitanio, A. I-Deamino-8-D-Arginine Vasopressin: A new pharmacological approach to the management of haemophilia and von Willebrand's disease. (1977). Lancet, 1, 869

9. Mannucci, P.M., Ruggeri, Z.M., Pareti, F.I. and Capitanio, A. (1977). DDAVP in haemophilia. Lancet, 2, 1171

10. Ludlam, C.A., Peake, I.R. Allen, N., Davies, B.L., Furlong, R.A. and Bloom, A.L. (1980). Factor VIII and fibrinolytic response to Deamino-8-D-Arginine Vasopressin in normal subjects and dissociate response in some patients with haemophilia and von Willebrand's disease. Br. J. Haemotol., 45, 499

11. Mannucci, P.M., Aberg, M., Nilsson, I.M. and Robertson, B. (1975). Mechanism of plasminogen activator and factor VIII increase after vaso-active drugs. Br. J. Haematol., 30, 81

12. Mannucci, P.M., Rota, L., Benvenuti, C. and Ruggeri, Z.M. (1979). Clinico-pharmacological studies of factor VIII response after DDAVP. Thrombosis Haemostasis, 42, 309

13. Nilsson, I.M. (1978). Report of the Working Party on factor VIII related antigens. Thrombosis Haemostasis, 39, 511

14. Mannucci, P.M., Pareti, F.I., Holmberg, L., Nilsson, I.M. and Ruggeri, Z.M. (1976). Studies on the prolonged bleeding time in von Willebrand's disease. J. Lab. Clin. Med., 88, 662

15. Schmitz-Huebner, U., Balleisen, L., Arenda, P., Pollman, H. and Sutor, A.H. (1980). DDAVP-induced changes of factor VIII-related activities and bleeding time in patients with von Willebrand's syndrome. Haemostasis, 9, 204

16. Lowe, G.D.O. Harvie, A., Forbes, C.D., Prentice, C.R.M. (1976). DDAVP in haemophilia. Br. Med. J., 4, 1110

17. Peake, I.R., Bloom, A.L., Giddings, J.C. and Ludlam, C.A. (1979). An immunoradiometric assay for procoagulant factor VIII antigen results in haemophilia, von Willebrand's disease and fetal plasma and serum. Br. J. Haematol., 42, 269

Discussion

Dr. Prentice: In our experience, the number of von Willebrands disease patients with relatively normal bleeding times and ristocetin co-factor levels above 5 per cent are very few compared to the number of the more severe types. Would you agree that in von Willebrands disease in general there may not be a major role for DDAVP because so few of them have this type of abnormality which is corrected by it.

Dr. Ludlam: In our experience most patients who have intermediate vWD with prolonged bleeding times do get a shortening even though they have quite low ristocetin co-factor activities it does seem to rise and they do get a shortening of bleeding times. I think there are a lot of patients, and it is not just confined to the group with the so-called autosomal haemophilia, who have the normal bleeding time but low ristocetin co-factor.

Prof. Stewart: What is a minor procedure?

Dr. Ludlam: It would depend whether one was the patient or the surgeon. Dental extraction, lymph node biopsies, sebaceous cysts, that sort of thing.

Dr. Leslie: The tachyphylaxis of the effect wearing off, when did the patient recover? Did it take a week, or six months? Could you go back to square one and get a good response again later, and if so how long did it take?

Dr. Ludlam: I do not know of any formal studies to look at this. My impression is it is probably about 2 days. Certainly I have given it to patients at daily intervals and have still seen the tachyphylaxis. Certainly when test doses are done before surgical procedures I would suggest they were more than 3 days before surgery.

Dr. Colvin: Discussing a minor procedure, on the rare occasions when I have taken tonsils out of children with vWD and I agreed to do so rather reluctantly, we have found that if they are given DDAVP for 24 hours in 2 or 3 doses with tranexamic acid, although that is a fairly major procedure, we have had no trouble at all with postoperative haemastasis, and I have reassured myself with the thought that I can actually see the tonsil fossa and if bleeding does occur I can give cryoprecipitate. So I have found it very useful in those circumstances, and I guess that is not such a minor procedure.

Dr. Ludlam: Dr. Colvin is probably right. I am just taking a conservative line.

Dr. Flute: Is there any evidence in the mild haemophiliac in particular, with 10 per cent levels, that the results are any better with DDAVP than they would be with tranexamic acid alone?

Dr. Ludlam: No. Not with DDAVP. We have done no clinical studies to look at the amount of bleeding. The number of patients we would have in any one year would make this a long study.

Prof. Bloom: I suppose it is reassuring to have a raised level of Factor VIII.

Dr. Ludlam: There are other studies that raise the Factor VIII level, but all the evidence suggests that this is the same Factor VIII, that is in the circulation.

10 Polyelectrolytes and preparation of Factor VIIIC

S. Middleton

Selective separation of proteins by chromatographic agents has been used extensively in plasma fractionation for many years. These agents include ion exhange groups on various types of solid phase matrices such as cellulose[1] and agarose[2]. In addition there has been recent emphasis on affinity chromatography[3] and on gel permeation chromatography for the separation of salt from protein on the basis of molecular size[4,5].

The advantages of these reagents such as increased resolution without denaturation and ease of solid liquid separations are thus well known.

A series of solid phase polyelectrolytes based on the copolymer ethylene maleic anhydride (EMA) has been developed for use in plasma fractionation[6]. The material is being employed in a production scale process for the preparation of human and porcine factor VIIIC for therapeutic use.

ETHYLENE MALEIC ANHYDRIDE POLYELECTROLYTE

The approximate stucture of the ethylene maleic anhydride polyelectrolyte or PE is shown in Figure 1.

The anhydride groups (x) are substituted with the positively charged dimethylamino-propylimide (DMAPI) groups (y).

The density of the positively charged group can be varied. For example, in PE E5 the PE is substituted with 5% DMAPI, whilst in PE 100, the PE is substituted with 100% DMAPI. Hydrolysis of the unreacted anhydride groups is prevented by the substitution of a non-reactive group.

0	5	10	15	20	30	50	70	100
E0	E5	E10	E15	E20	E30	E50	E70	E100

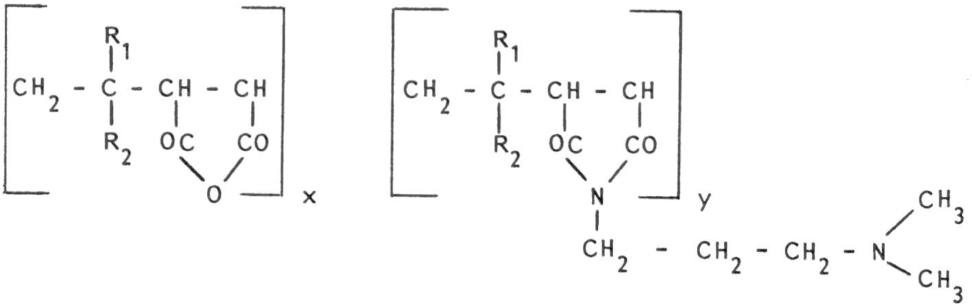

$$\left[CH_2 - \underset{\underset{R_2}{|}}{\overset{\overset{R_1}{|}}{C}} - \underset{\underset{O}{\diagdown O \diagup}}{\overset{|}{CH}} - \underset{CO}{\overset{|}{CH}} \right]_x \qquad \left[CH_2 - \underset{\underset{R_2}{|}}{\overset{\overset{R_1}{|}}{C}} - \underset{\underset{N}{OC}}{\overset{|}{CH}} - \underset{CO}{\overset{|}{CH}} \right]_y$$

$$CH_2 - CH_2 - CH_2 - N \diagup^{CH_3}_{\diagdown CH_3}$$

x = Number of repeating units of basic polymer
y = Number of repeating units of DMAPI

Figure 1   Approximate structure of ethylene maleic anhydride polyelectrolyte
approximate mole percentage dimethylamino-propylimide (DMAPI)

Adsorption and elution of proteins to the PE is primarily achieved through electrostatic binding to the cationic imide group. Thus the most important parameters affecting protein separation in this system, are those which affect the electrostatic charge on the protein or the PE.

FRACTIONATION OF HUMAN PLASMA USING PE

By adjustment of pH, ionic strength and charge density on the PE, a total fractionation system for human plasma has been developed (Figure 2).

Each step may be used independently or supplementary to other fractionation procedures, such as the Cohn ethanol fractionation[7].

Adsorption and elution of protein can be achieved in a batch or column mode and the PE separated readily from the supernatant liquor by centifugation or filtration.

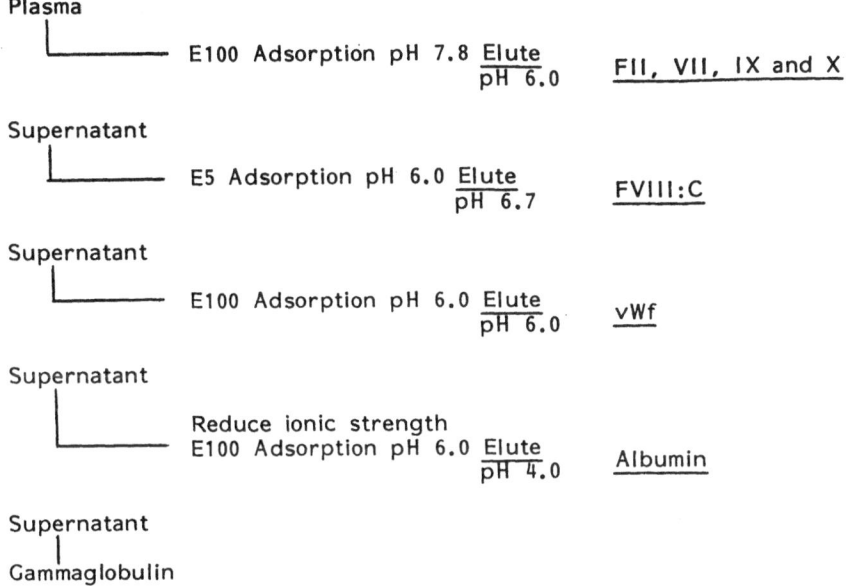

Figure 2   Basic polyelectrolyte fractionation scheme.   A.J. Johnson,
            et al. (1978)

FACTORS II, VII, IX and X

The prothrombin complex, Factors II, VII, IX and X, consists of moderate size proteins, about 75,000 m.w. with an acidic pH[8]. They are strongly adsorbed to the essentially basic PE E100 at pH 7.8 and can then be eluted, by increasing the ionic strength of the medium and by lowering the charge on the protein by the reduction of the pH to 6.0.

ALBUMIN

Albumin and the alpha – and beta – globulins including fibrinogen are bound to the PE E100 at a low ionic strength at pH 6.0. At this pH, both PE and proteins are highly charged. By washing the PE at pH 5.0 most of the contaminating proteins are eluted. Albumin is recovered at pH 4.0 below its isoelectric point.

GAMMAGLOBULIN

Since the isoelectric point of gammaglobulin is high, it is not adsorbed to the PE. It can thus be recovered in a purified state from the supernatant, after adsorption of the albumin and alpha – and beta – globulins, on PE E100.

FACTOR VIIIC

The isoelectric point of Factor VIII is undoubtedly in the acid range, facilitating the adsorption of this protein on the high or low charge density PE's. Adsorption is optimal at pH 6.0 where the PE is maximally protonated. It is found, however, that elution of the Factor VIII is difficult, requiring a high ionic strength and a low charge density PE, possibly to reduce the number of bonds between the PE and the high molecular weight protein. It has been observed that the use of a NaCl concentration greater than 1.5 mol/l actually inhibits elution, and, it is possible that there is some hydrophobic bond formation between the Factor VIII and the PE in addition to the electrostatic bonds.

VON WILLEBRAND FACTOR ACTIVITY

It has been found that while Factor VIIIC is adsorbed to the low charge density PE, the Factor VIII related antigen and ristocetin co-factor activity require the more highly charged PE E100 or conditions of reduced ionic strength for adsorption. Elution is carried out at increased ionic strength with a buffer containing 0.75 mol/l NaCl.

THERAPEUTIC PREPARATIONS OF HUMAN FACTOR VIIIC AND VON WILLEBRAND FACTOR

The fractionation of the Factor VIII complex suggests that the possibility exists of achieving two types of concentrate. A concentrate of Factor VIIIC for the treatment of haemophiliacs and a concentrate of von Willebrand factor for the treatment of von Willebrand's disease, thus making more efficient use of the existing Factor VIII pool.

These types of concentrate are completely novel and their efficacy in vivo remains to be established. In collaboration with The Blood Products Laboratory, Elstree, a concentrate of Factor VIIIC has been prepared and is presently being assessed in vivo. In addition, development work is underway to prepare a concentrate of von Willebrand factor.

As can be seen, relatively low amounts of protein are adsorbed to the PE and extensive washing with 0.35 mol/l NaCl has resulted in a very low recovery of porcine protein. In contrast the Factor VIIIC is almost totally adsorbed. The yield of Factor VIIIC in this high purity preparation tends to be low, but by adjusting the volume and ionic strength of the wash it is possible to achieve higher or lower levels of purity, with correspondingly lower or higher yields, depending on the type of concentrate required.

Table 2 shows the fractionation of the Factor VIII complex that is achieved using polyelectrolyte.

Table 2.   Fractionation of the Factor VIII complex (FVIIIC, FVIIIRAG and PAF) during PE processing

n = 4	% Recovery from intermediate purity FVIII		
	FVIIIC	FVIIIRAG	PAF
E5 supernatant	2.6 ± 1.3	72.9 ± 25.0	70 ± 23.0
Lyophilised PEG concentrate	14.3 ± 3.0	2.0 ± 1.0	0.85 ± 0.60

FVIIIC	=	Human units
FVIIIRAG	=	Porcine units
FVIIIPAF	=	Porcine units

Table 3.   Comparative levels of FVIIIC and PAF

n = 4	FVIIIC (U/ml)	PAF (U/ml)	Ratio FVIIIC : PAF
Plasma	5	1	5
Cryoprecipitate	36.3 ± 7.3	2.20 ± 0.76	18.7 ± 6.1
Lyophilised PEG concentrate	33.1 ± 7.1	0.1 ± 0	331 ± 71

FVIIIC	=	Human units
FVIIIPAF	=	Porcine units

As can be seen, while the Factor VIIIC is almost totally adsorbed, the Factor VIIIRAG and the PAF remain in the supernatant, a relatively low level of the Factor VIIIRAG and the PAF being recovered in the final product. This is further shown in Table 3 where the ratio of factor VIIIC to PAF is illustrated.

Essentially the ratio of Factor VIIIC to PAF is increased over 18-fold during the polyelectrolyte procedure.

IN VIVO RECOVERY BY INFUSION INTO VON WILLEBRAND PIG

In order to determine the in vivo response of this type of material, porcine Factor VIIIC has been injected by Dr. Helen Lee into two von Willebrand pigs with the co-operation of Dr. Bowie at the Mayo Clinic (Figure 4).

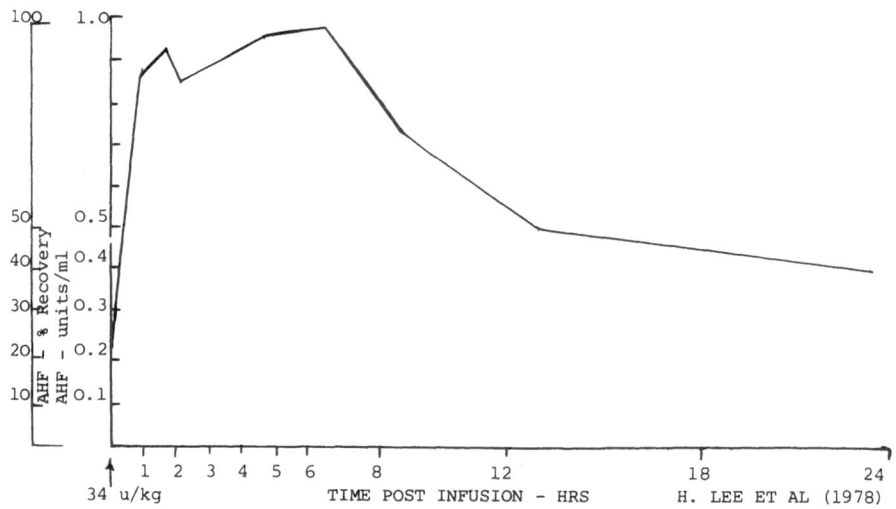

Figure 4   Infusion of 34 U/kg of porcine Factor VIIIC in a pig with
von Willebrand's disease showing recovery (90%), T1/2
life (9 hours)

After infusing 34 U/kg, the coagulant activity rose from 0.2 U/ml to a peak of 0.93 U/ml, giving a recovery of approximately 90% of the expected value. It remained at this level for 6 hours and then gradually decreased to the pre-infusion level at 24 hours. The half disappearance time was approximately 9 hours.

SUMMARY

Solid phase polyelectrolytes offer a simple, non–denaturing and flexible procedure for the fractionation of animal and human plasma. Using PE's it is possible to fractionate the Factor VIIIC complex to obtain concentrates of Factor VIIIC and von Willebrand factor for clinical use. The polyelectrolytes are being used at a production scale for the preparation of concentrated porcine Factor VIIIC that is virtually free of PAF. This type of preparation has already been used with success and no clinically significant thrombocytopenia or other serious side–effects were observed.

REFERENCES

1. Middleton, S.M., Bennett, I.H. and Smith J.K. (1973). A therapeutic concentrate of coagulation factors II, IX and X from citrated FVIII depleted plasma. Vox Sang., 24, 441

2. Haystek, J., Brummelhuis, H.G.J. and Krijnen, H.W. (1973). Contributions to the optimal use of Human Blood. 11 The large scale preparation of prothrombin complex. A comparison between two methods using the anion exchangers DEAE cellulose DE52 and DEAE Sephadex A-50. Vox Sang., 25, 113

3. Miller-Anderson, M., Borg, H. and Andersson L-O., (1974). Purification of Antithrombin III by affinity chromatography. Thromb. Res., 5, 439

4. Curling, J.M., Berglof, J., Lindquist I-0, and Eriksson, S. (1977). A chromatographic procedure for the purification of human plasma albumin. Vox Sang., 33, 97

5. Friedli, H. and Kistler, P. (1972). Removal of ethanol from albumin by gel filtration in the manufacturing of human serum albumin solutions for clinical use. Clinica, 26, 25

6. Johnson, A.J., MacDonald, V.E., Semar, M., Fields, J.E., Schuck, J., Lewis, C. and Brind, J. (1978). Preparation of the major plasma fractions by solid phase polyelectrolytes. J. Lab. Clin. Med., 92, 194

7. Cohn, E.J., Strang, L.E., Hughes, W.L., Mulford, D.J., Ashforth,

J.M., Malin, M. and Taylor, H.L. (1946). Preparation and properties of serum and plasma proteins. I.V. A system for the separation into fractions of the protein and lipoprotein components of biological tissues and fluids. J. Am. Chem. Soc., 68, 459

8. Davie, E.W. and Fujikaura, K. (1975). Mechanisms of blood coagulation. Ann. Rev. Biochem., 44, 799

9. Bidwell, E. (1955). The purification of antihaemophilic globulin from animal blood. Br. J. Haematol., 1, 386

10. MacFarlane, E.G., Mallam P.C., Withs, L.J., Bidwell, E., Biggs, R., Fraenkel, G.J., Honey, G.Z. and Taylor, K.B. (1957). Surgery in haemophilia. The use of animal antihaemophilic globulin and human plasma in thirteen cases. Lancet, 2, 25

11. Lilley, P.A., Kernoff, P.B.A. and Tuddenham, E.G.D. (1978). Clinical experience with a new porcine FVIII concentrate. Congress of the World Federation of Haemophilia XIII

12. Donadio, D., Allain, J.P., Rouanet, C., Navarro, M. and Izarn, P. (1978). The use of porcine FVIII and plasmapheresis in the treatment of a patient with a high titre antibody to FVIII (1978). 17th Congress International Society of Haematology and Blood Transfusion

13. Forbes, C.D. and Prentice, C.R.M. (1973). Aggregation of human platelets by purified porcine and bovine antihaemophilic factor. Nature New Biol., 241, 149

Discussion

Dr. Crawford: I have been trying to find out something about these polyelectrolytes for some time. Is the supply situation better than it was said to be?

Mrs. Middleton: At present we have all this particular polyelectrolyte and it is not freely available yet.

Dr. Crawford: Secondly, what are the prospects for human factors? Could something better than the NHS intermediate Factor VIII be made by the polyelectrolyte technology?

Mrs. Middleton: As I said, we are presently trying to make a concentrate of Factor VIIIC with the Blood Products Laboratory – and we are testing it. We have produced some.

Dr. Ludlam: Can I ask what stabilises the Factor VIIIC in your bottles of it?

Mrs. Middleton: There is no stabiliser.

Dr. Ludlam: Just Factor VIIIC alone?

Mrs. Middleton: Factor VIIIC in albumin. That is all there is. It is very stable. It is stable on the bench for 48 hours in the liquid state and there is no loss of Factor VIIIC. This is the porcine material.

Prof. Stewart: One of the problems of the old porcine material was that patients became immunised to it in 4 to 8 days. In other words, they got no response after that time. Am I to understand that Dr. Kernoff's patients do not become immunised?

Dr. Kernoff: One aspect of the phenomenon is this business of resistance, which was seen in the old days when porcine material was given to patients without inhibitors, and then they developed this but did not have any measurable inhibitor. It is a very interesting theoretical problem, but I do not know that we can crack it now, because we are really at this moment only talking about porcine for use in patients who have definitely got inhibitors.

All I can say is that in the courses we gave, we saw no particular evidence of anything resembling that phenomenon. When a patient did get a circulating Factor VIII level he continued to get it, but then only one course was given for up to 7 days or so. Most of the courses we gave were much shorter than that, and what we are trying to do now is to titrate the dose down and use smaller and smaller doses just to see how short a course we can get away with.

Prof. Bloom: This question was put to me some time ago by Dr. Rizza. We wondered whether these patients treated with porcine product would develop an antibody, not so much to VIIIC but to the aggregation factor. Are you following the ristocetin co-factor activity in your patients to see if they develop an anti-ristocetin co-factor?

Dr. Kernoff: We shall be following everything. I can give assurances of that. I think that it is around that area that this whole business of resistance may revolve. There was some suggestion that patients would develop antibodies to Factor VIII related antigen or something, and that complex would be removed from the circulation which accounts for resistance. But it is an interesting thought. Whether it will be of clinical relevance one really cannot know.

Prof. Bloom: Although I accept that you are separating these off by 99.99 per cent nevertheless, there may be a little bit of immunogenic PAF left, so this could be a point.

11

Oral administration of Factor VIII in lipid vesicles

H. C. Hemker and R. F. A. Zwaal

The prevention or treatment of severe bleedings in patients with haemophilia A presently depends on intravenous administration of partially purified preparations of the missing coagulation Factor VIII. In spite of the revolutionary breakthrough that came in the treatment of haemophiliacs with the introduction of suitable Factor VIII preparations for clinical use, this therapy still presents a variety of problems, not the least of them being the recurrent injections themselves. Oral administration of these Factor VIII preparations is useless due to extensive degradation of the protein in the gastrointestinal tract. This breakdown may be overcome to a certain extent if the protein is packed in liposomes, which may decrease exposure to the digestive proteolytic enzymes. It has been reported that liposome entrapped proteins are capable of entering intact cells[1], and insulin loaded liposomes administered orally to diabetic rats can cause a fall in the blood glucose level[2].

FACTOR VIII LOADED LIPOSOMES

Liposomes are artificial structures of multilamellar concentric bilayers of phospholipids that form spontaneously upon suspending lipids in water[3]. When liposomes are prepared in the presence of aqueous solution of a protein, 5-15% of the protein may become entrapped in the interstices between the bilayers[4]. Because Factor VIII has been reported to interact hydrophobically with phospholipids[5], we thought that it might be possible to preferentially absorb Factor VIII on phospholipids and therefore obtain liposomes with a much higher Factor VIII content than is usually obtained with non-lipid binding proteins. In spite of the fact that liposomes and their entrapped proteins are also susceptible to gastrointestinal breakdown, we thought that the specific binding of Factor VIII to the lipids and the much higher protein loading of the liposome, would produce an increased resistance to proteolytic attack and improve the chances for the protein to reach the target undamaged.

The preparations to be used for oral administration were made from egg yolk lecithin containing 5-10% of phosphatidic acid and solutions of either Factor VIII concentrate or cryoprecipitate. Usually 50 mg of phospholipid were used per ml of Factor VIII solution. A detailed description of the procedure has been published[6].

The fraction of non-entrapped protein can be measured in the supernatant after centrifuging the liposomes at 50,000 x g for 10 minutes. This fluid contained 19-32% of the original Factor VIII added and usually more than 80% of the fibrinogen present in Factor VIII preparations. This strongly suggests that the liposome preparations are indeed preferentially enriched with Factor VIII, presumably due to the strong interaction between Factor VIII and the lipids. Direct measurement of the entrapped protein has so far been hampered by the presence of phospholipids. It is not to be expected, however, that significant denaturation of Factor VIII occurs because carrying out the same manipulations with a Factor VIII solution in the absence of lipids causes less than 5% inactivation.

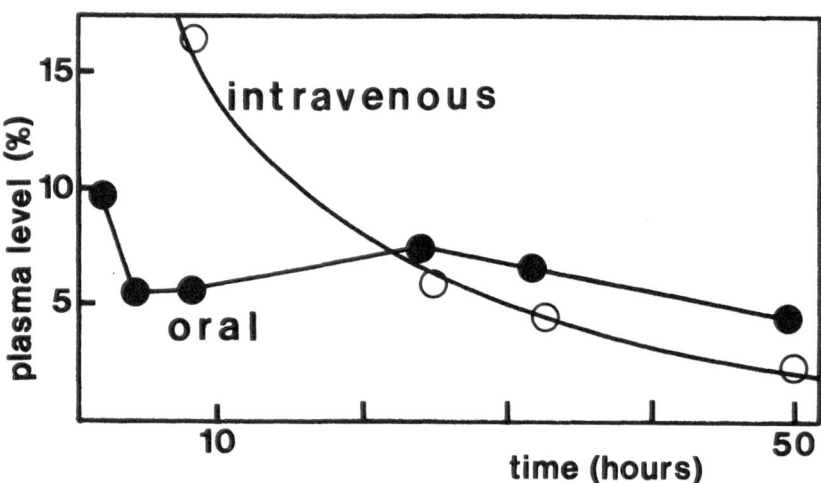

Figure 1   Factor VIII activity in plasma after oral and intravenous administration of Factor VIII to a patient with severe haemophilia. Concentrations were determined according to Veltkamp[7] and are expressed as a percentage of Factor VIII concentration in pooled normal plasma (n = 30)

Each sample was tested 4 times. SEM did not exceed 9% of value observed. At zero time 800 units of Factor VIII were given orally or intravenously. Factor VIII concentration in the untreated subject is less than 0.5% of normal. Concentration after intravenous administration measured before 9 hours were between 30% and 15% and have been omitted from the graph.

ORAL ADMINISTRATION

In a first experiment Factor VIII loaded liposomes were given before breakfast to a patient with severe haemophilia A (mean Factor VIII level when not on treatment less than 0.5% of normal; no circulating antibodies). The results are shown in Figure 1. Plasma levels after intravenous administration of the same amount of Factor VIII (not entrapped in liposomes) are also shown. The patient had haematuria before ingestion of the liposome preparation; this disappeared on the day of the experiment and returned 3 days thereafter. Plasma Factor VIII activity did not rise when either liposomes or Factor VIII were given separately. Some of the Factor VIII administered in the liposomes appeared in the plasma as Factor VIII activity. This activity, though much lower than observed shortly after intravenous administration, persisted for some 50 hours. This suggests that orally administered Factor VIII does not enter the plasma directly but is liberated from an as yet unknown depot.

Repeating the experiment with the same patient produced similar results, but variable results were obtained with different patients (Table 1). Of the 6 patients (all without circulating antibodies), 2 patients showed a significant and prophylactic increase of some 10% although the time period required to reach this level varied. In 2 patients only a minor increase was observed whereas treatment was ineffective with 2 other patients. It is to be noted that in no instance could any significant increase in serum phospholipid concentration be detected. This suggests that the Factor VIII containing liposomes do not enter the blood as such, which may limit the chances for new antibodies to form.

DISCUSSION

Although it is hardly possible to draw conclusions from

comparable to, or even longer than, that observed after intravenous administration of the same amount of Factor VIII. We have no explanation for the fact that some patients show little or no response. The efficacy of the treatment will certainly depend upon protection from, and time of exposure to, proteolytic digestion in the gastrointestinal tract. In this respect it is of interest that upon oral administration of insulin loaded liposomes to fasted and non-fasted rats, we only observed a large drop in blood glucose level in the group of fasted rats (Figure 2). A difference in resorption time may be responsible for this effect. Whether or not the resistance to digestive enzymes can also be improved by altering the phospholipid composition still needs to be investigated.

Table 1   Oral administration of 1300 U Factor VIII concentrate, trapped in 7 g liposomes (PC : PA = 9 : 1)

Patients	F VIII % t = o	Maximal F VIII % t = x
1	0.7	10.0 (x = 1.5 h)
2	3.8	10.2 (x = 4 h)
3	0.5	1.4 (x = 2 h)
4	0.6	1.2 (x = 2 h)
5	5.0	no change in 5 h
6	0.6	no change in 5 h

Patients 4-6 did not receive the material on an empty stomach.

We conclude that oral administration of Factor VIII in liposomes can lead to therapeutic plasma levels of Factor VIII, although the circumstances required for a successful treatment are not yet completely understood. A more extensive investigation is required in which particular attention should be paid to possible undesired antigenic reactions, although at present we have no indications that these occur.

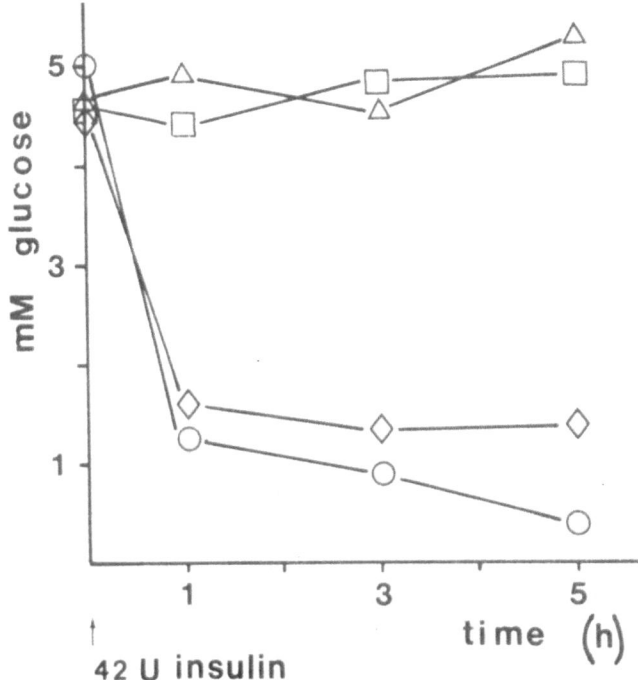

Figure 2   Plasma levels of glucose after oral administration of liposome entrapped insulin to fasted and non-fasted rats. —☐-☐—, non-fasted rats; –◇-◇— , fasted rats; —△-△— , non-entrapped insulin; —○-○- , intraperitoneal administration of non-entrapped insulin

ACKNOWLEDGEMENT

We thank Dr. J.W. ten Cate, Wilhelmina Gasthuis, Amsterdam, for his co-operation in studying a number of his patients.

REFERENCES

1.   Gregoriadis, G., Siliprandi, N. and Turchetto, E. (1977). Possible implications in the use of exogenous phospholipids. Life Sci., **20**, 1773

2.   Patel, H.M. and Ryman, B.E. (1976). Oral administration of insulin by encapsulation within liposomes. FEBS letters, **62**, 60

3. Bangham, A.D., Standish, M.M. and Weissmann, G. (1965). The action of steroids and streptolysin S on the permeability of phospholipid structures to cations. J. Mol. Biol., 13, 253

4. Sessa, G. and Weissmann, G. (1970). Incorporation of lysozyme into liposomes. A model for structure-linked latency. J. Biol. Chem., 245, 3295

5. Hemker, H.C. and Kahn, M.J.P. (1967). The reaction sequence of blood coagulation. Nature, 215, 1201

6. Hemker, H.C., Hermens, W.Th., Muller A.D. and Zwaal, R.F.A. (1980). Oral treatment of haemophilia A by gastrointestinal absorption of factor VIII entrapped in liposomes. Lancet, i, 70

7. Veltkamp, J.J., Drion, E.F. and Loeliger, E.A. (1968). Detection of the carrier state in hereditary coagulation disorders. Thromb. Diath. Haemorrh., 19, 279

Discussion

Dr. Austen: Could Professor Zwaal tell us how he knows he has got so much Factor VIII entrapped in the liposome. I believe he stated 60-80 per cent. We have been preparing these liposomes over a long period now and my figure is nearer 1 per cent, which is rather different. Incidentally, we have treated one Factor IX deficient patient and two rabbits so far, with a total failure on all counts.

Prof. Zwaal: Had we studied patient No. 6 first, we would probably have dropped the whole thing. It was just a matter of luck that we hit the right patient or the good patients first.

I do not know what Dr. Austen's phospholipid composition is. It is absolutely necessary to have a negative surface charge. Normally we use Ac-lecithin containing about 10 per cent phosphoteric acid, or in between 5 and 10 per cent, and the negative surface charge is required for Factor VIII to bind to the phospholipd. It does not spontaneously bind to pure lecithin. The other question - how do we measure the entrapment? There are two ways. There is the very easy way of spinning down liposomes and measuring how much is left in the supernatant. That is a very easy way of doing it. The more complicated way is when one wants to know how much is really entrapped. In other words, what is not measured in the supernatant, is that really entrapped, or is that denatured. Initial experiments in which we have degraded the liposomes, with phospholipases, show indeed that the total procedure to prepare the liposomes does not result in a loss that is more than 5 per cent of the Factor VIII activity. So where liposomes are degraded with phospholipases, Factor VIII can be measured because it is again released and the amount that was entrapped can be measured.

Dr. Austen: So that in fact one can take the liposomes, get zero Factor VIII in an assay, then lyse these liposomes, and in the following assay get 60 per cent of the starting material.

Prof. Zwaal: That is correct.

Prof. Stewart: Does it make any difference what sort of Factor VIII preparation is used?

Prof. Zwaal: We have tried two preparations, the cryoprecipitate and the Factor VIII concentrate.

Prof. Stewart: What concentrate?

Prof. Zwaal: I think it was Swiss in origin but I am not quite sure.

Prof. Stewart: Does it make any difference?

Prof. Zwaal: No. Not in these experiments — at least in the first patients, who always respond successfully.

Dr. Ludlam: Has Prof. Zwaal tried the control experiment giving the liposomes without Factor VIII and then measuring the Factor VIII level in the blood?

Prof. Zwaal: Of course we have. The result is nil.

Dr. Tuddenham: What sort of recovery does Prof. Zwaal get? How much Factor VIII does he put into the vessel in which he prepared the liposomes and how much gets into the patient?

Prof. Zwaal: Assuming a trap of between 60 and 80 per cent when we introduce 1300 units of Factor VIII. These are really entrapped units, so we started with approximately 1700 or 1800 units of Factor VIII of which about 1300 units were entrapped. But the first experiment was done with 800 units.

Dr. Tuddenham: How much got into the patient?

Prof. Zwaal: We have not really measured that. The therapeutic level above 5 per cent is maintained for at least the same time or longer than the level reached with an intravenous injection.

Dr. Pepper: As Prof. Zwaal states, specific entrapment is usually rather inefficient, and 60 per cent does imply some kind of specific affinity. Is there any other evidence, apart from those numbers, of the nature of the interaction which you postulated between VIIIC and the phospholipids in this situation?

Prof. Zwaal: Normally given pure labelled Factor VIII, one can do binding constants between Factor VIII and phospholipids. As I stated, this depends on the negative surface charge which is very similar to Factor V.

Dr. Pepper: Is it reported by anybody else in this sort of situation?

Prof. Zwaal: That there is a binding of Factor VIII in the lipids? I think there are a number of indications from the literature, but as far as I can recall there is no separate article devoted to that.

Prof. Bloom: Dr. Pepper is asking whether Prof. Hemker has repeated his earlier experiments with the use of phospholipids that they are actually using in the liposomes.

Prof. Zwaal: No, he has not. But I showed very early experiments. But, when we take the pure Factor VIII preparations as are presently being prepared, we can label them and measure binding between these Factor VIII and the lipids, and we find only high affinity when the lipid is negatively charged.

Dr. Birch: How stable are liposomal preparations because in practical terms if they are not likely to prove stable on the bench or in the refrigerator for some time, they may not be of much use.

Prof. Zwaal: Normally a liposome preparation is stable when it is not sterilised for about 2 to 3 days in a refrigerator. It might be interesting to look at whether one can lyophyllise the complete liposomal preparation, or just freeze it and see whether it can be used again without any loss of activity in the Factor VIII. But this has not been done. Normally the preparation is stable for about 2 to 3 days.

Dr. Delamore: Has anyone tried giving it with the appropriate lipolytic enzymes to see whether that will promote absorption?

Prof. Zwaal: Why should one promote absorption?

Dr. Delamore: Prof. Zwaal did suggest that if it was not given on a fasting stomach he did not get the appropriate action from lipolytic enzymes.

Prof. Zwaal: The idea behind it is very simple, that there is an enhanced degradation due to the production of lipolytic enzymes when the stomach is not empty. But one can simply degrade the liposomes by lipolytic enzymes. Of course one can. And then the Factor VIII is liberated.

Prof. Bloom: Then presumably it would not get absorbed. Can Prof. Zwaal postulate the mechanisms of absorption?

Prof. Zwaal: I have no idea. I can speculate on it. It has been shown that normally most of the lecithin which is administered orally is degraded, and the fatty acids of the lecithin appear for instance in triglycerides in the blood. It has also been shown that under certain conditions lecithin can be taken up completely as a complete molecule. But in this case we have measured the possibility of a rise in the serum levels of lecithin in the plasma and we could not detect any, whereas we could have when most of the lecithin would have been liberated to the plasma.

Prof. Bloom: Presumably this goes into the portal system, into the chyle. Does it get a deposit there in the lymph nodes?

Prof. Zwaal: The fact that it is maintained, at least in the successful experiments, for about 3 days at a level of between 5 and 10 per cent simply suggests that it is liberated from a depot as yet unknown.

Prof. Bloom: Which is why I asked whether the depot could possibly be in the lymphatic system.

Prof. Zwaal: It could be. It could be anywhere.

Dr. Preston: Has there been an opportunity to test the liposomes in patients with vW disease?

Prof. Zwaal: That is a very good question. We are really willing to do this, but as I mentioned this is only a very small sideline in our laboratory. We do not normally do research into haemophilia.

Prof. Bloom: This is a very exciting possibility. I really hope that it does develop.

12

Use of activated prothrombin complex in Factor VIII inhibitors

C. F. Abildgaard

Because the development of activated prothrombin complex concentrates (PCC) for use in the treatment of bleeding in patients with inhibitors to Factor VIII has been a topic associated with controversy and confusion, I will begin with a brief review. The materials used in the United States are listed in Table 1.

Table 1. Prothrombin complex concentrates used for treatment of Factor VIII inhibitors in the U.S.

"Activated"	Regular
Autofactor IX (Hyland) (spontaneous)	KONYNE (Cutter)
Autoplex (Hyland) (controlled)	PROPLEX (Hyland)
FEIBA (Immuno)	

In 1972 Fekete and co-workers at Hyland described their use of an activated PCC to treat a patient with haemophilia complicated by an inhibitor to Factor VIII[1]. The material in this study was a spontaneously activated form of Proplex (Hyland) which was subsequently made available as an investigational material (Autofactor IX). In 1974 Kurczynski and Penner reported their experience using this material for the treatment of a number of bleeding episodes in patients with inhibitors[2] and considerable interest in this approach to treatment developed in many centres.

My first experience with this approach was in 1975 when I was faced with the problem of treating a 12 year old boy with a high level of inhibitor for a massive abdominal haemorrhage that followed minor trauma. No response was observed during the first 48 hours when he received 20,000 units Factor VIII/24 hours as a constant infusion. A small amount of Autofactor IX was obtained and three infusions (16 bottles) were given in an 8 hour period. Although there was initial relief of pain, stabilisation of abdominal girth, and decrease in the partial thromboplastin time (PTT), by the following day his symptoms were worse.

At the suggestion of Dr. Aaron Josephson, further treatment was given using a regular PCC, Konyne (Cutter) being the one available at that time in our hospital. The administration of Konyne (80 U/kg) was followed by significant shortening of the PTT and clinical improvement. Three days later, clinical evidence of further bleeding recurred which improved after additional Konyne administration. Again 48 hours later there was recurrent bleeding with extension into the left hemithorax. The patient was then treated with daily infusions for 7 days. The haemorrhage stopped and the massive soft tissue haematoma gradually resolved over the next 4 weeks.

In view of this remarkable response in a patient with a life-threatening haemorrhage, we began to use Konyne in other patients with inhibitors, reporting results of this experience in 1976[3]. This report included the treatment of 64 episodes in 5 patients using Konyne in doses from 15 to 100 Factor IX U/kg. I review this early experience to emphasise several points of interest related to the effect of treatment on the PTT:

1. With both Autofactor IX and Konyne, correction of the PTT was to normal or near normal levels following the administration of doses of 80 to 100 U/kg.

2. The observed shortening of the PTT sometimes persisted for 12-24 hours.

3. The degree of shortening of the PTT observed varied, depending on the partial thromboplastin reagent used to perform the test.

4. As bleeding episodes were treated earlier with smaller doses of Konyne, little or no decrease in the PTT was observed despite clinical efficacy of the therapy.

Other investigators have described successful use of PCC in the treatment of inhibitors with over 400 episodes in 57 patients reported in the literature[4-13]. This experience includes the use of both activated PCC (Autoplex) and regular commercially available PCC (Konyne-Cutter and Proplex-Hyland). We continued to use Konyne routinely for this purpose and were able to manage patients with Factor VIII inhibitors in the same fashion as those without inhibitors. Bleeding was treated early with doses of Factor IX no greater than those used for similar problems in Factor IX deficient patients. However, by late 1976 we became aware of a change in the efficacy of standard PCC in the treatment of bleeding in patients with inhibitors. This change was first brought to our attention by a patient who had been receiving successful early treatment with Konyne for nearly 2 years. He informed us that the treatment was no longer effective. On subsequent infusions using larger doses, we observed no change in the PTT and other patients noted a decrease in efficacy. This curious change in the efficacy of Konyne and Proplex has been observed by other investigators and has been confirmed by the results of a double blind study in the U.S.[14]. The study was a multicentre double trial of Konyne, Proplex or albumin placebo for the treatment of early haemarthroses. The batches of PCC were produced in 1977 and the study was performed during 1978-79. Fifty-one patients were entered in the study and 149 treatment episodes were analysed (Konyne - 53, Proplex - 45, placebo - 51). In short, approximately 50% of those treated with Konyne or Proplex had a favourable response at 6 hours, compared to 25% of those receiving the placebo.

As mentioned earlier, the initial Autofactor IX consisted of spontaneously activated lots of Proplex. Although the active principle of this material in bypassing Factor VIII to promote haemostasis in vivo remains unknown, it has been possible to develop a reproducible controlled activated product. The remainder of this report will deal with the use of such a material currently licensed in the U.S. as anti-inhibitor coagulant complex or Autoplex. This product became available for investigation in 1977 and the experience to be reported is that accumulated by myself, Dr. John Penner in Ann Arbor, Michigan and our co-workers[15]. The studies include 14 patients with severe Factor VIII deficiency complicated by inhibitors of which all but one were high responders. Of 25 minor bleeding episodes treated, 16 were haemarthroses and the responses are shown in Table 2.

Table 2   Haemarthroses (16) treated with Autoplex (23-80 U/kg)

	8 hr	24 hr	48 hr
PAIN relief	8	6	2
range of motion	5	8	3

Nine other minor bleeding episodes were treated as shown in Table 3.

Table 3   Other MINOR bleeds (9) treated with Autoplex. (39 - 105 U/kg)

	8 hr	24 hr	48 hr
pain, swelling or cessation of bleeding	6	2	1

The response of all 25 minor bleeding episodes in relation to dose of Autoplex is shown in Table 4.

Table 4   Response to Autoplex in all MINOR bleeds (25)

DOSE	RESPONSE			
	Exc.	Good	Fair	Poor
< 50 U/kg	1	3	3	0
> 50 U/kg	13	5	0	0

There were no failures and the three fair responses were in patients who received less than 50 U/kg. To illustrate the importance of dose in relation to the type of bleeding I will describe one case in more detail. A 17 year old patient with a high responding inhibitor fell and struck his cheek on a bath tub. When seen approximately 12 hours later, there was a walnut-sized haematoma in his cheek and he was treated with 50

U/kg of Autoplex. Twenty-four hours later the bleed had progressed to include the entire cheek. Following a second dose of Autoplex (100 U/kg), the bleed stopped promptly and resolved without further treatment.

The ten major bleeding episodes treated with Autoplex include the following:

CLOSED

    Epidural

    Tongue, floor of mouth

    Groin, retroperitoneal

    Massive retroperitoneal

OPEN

    Puncture wound under tongue

    Laceration, forearm

    Multiple lacerations

    Multiple fractures and lacerations

    Total hip replacement

    Resection of pseudotumour

The epidural haemorrhage occurred in a 6 year old boy who fell from a slide. He suffered a basilar skull fracture and a fractured clavicle and was lethargic on admission. Computerised tomography revealed an epidural haemorrhage. He received Autoplex 100 U/kg every 8-12 hours for 14 days, then daily for 3 days. The lethargy improved within 12 hours and there was eventual complete resolution of the epidural haemorrhage by CT scan. Hypofibrinogenaemia occurred on day 3 (284 mg/dl to 84 mg/dl) and on day 13 (158 mg/dl to 73 mg/dl) with normal platelets, Factor V and euglobulin lysis time and negative tests for fibrin monomer and fibrin degradation products. The episodes of hypofibrinogenaemia were treated with cryoprecipitate and were not associated with further clinical problems.

Since this experience others have reported the successful use of Autoplex in treating central nervous system haemorrhage[16]. This experience contrasts with a 1960 series of 14 non-inhibitor patients with subdural or epidural bleeding with 11 deaths[17].

The two patients subjected to major surgery were treated by Dr. Penner in Michigan. Initial increased inhibitor levels were decreased by plasmapheresis and Factor VIII concentrate was used for the first 6 days until anamnestic responses occurred. Autoplex was then used to maintain haemostasis for 20 days in the patient with the hip replacement and over 30 days in the patient with resection of a large pseudotumour.

The most recent experience with massive trauma occurred in a 19 year old who was in an auto accident suffering a closed fracture of his right femur, penetrating wound of an elbow, deep laceration of the forehead and intraperitoneal bleeding due to torn omentum. Because his initial inhibitor level was only 4 Bethesda units, initial treatment was with constant infusion Factor VIII (135,000 units over 6 days), followed by Autoplex 100 U/kg every 8 to 24 hours (182,000 units from day 6 to 24). Despite these multiple serious injuries, his course has been satisfactory. His inhibitor level increased to 70 Bethesda units by the seventh day.

As a result of this experience, our current recommendations for treatment of bleeding in patients with inhibitors is summarised in Table 5.

Table 5   Recommendations for treatment of patients with Factor VIII inhibitors

Type of patient	MINOR bleed	MAJOR bleed
Low responder (less than 5 Bethesda units)	Factor VIII	Factor VIII
High responder with less than 5 Bethesda units	Activated PCC	Factor VIII until anamestic response, then activated PCC
High responder with greater than 5 Bethesda units	Activated PCC	Activated PCC

At the present time recommendations for Autoplex dose are as follows:

Early or minimal bleed	25 U/kg
Minor bleed	50 U/kg
Major (life-threatening) bleed	100 U/kg (repeated every 6-24 hours as indicated)

In addition to the experience with Autoplex, we have treated 15 episodes of haemarthroses with FEIBA (50 U/kg) during the past few months and all have responded with a single infusion, but we have had little experience using FEIBA for more serious bleeding episodes.

There are a number of unsolved problems relating to the use of activated PCC for the treatment of inhibitors including:

1. Unknown mechanism of action interfering with:
   a) Assay of product
   b) Ability to determine recovery and survival of the active principle in patients.
2. Excessive cost of therapy
3. Concern regarding potential untoward side-effects

Although the latter have not been observed with Autoplex, there have been significant thrombotic complications described following the use of the large doses of regular PCC in a few patients with inhibitors[14].

In an attempt to compare present products, we have performed some preliminary in vitro studies. Two or three lots of three regular PCC and three activated PCC (Autoplex, FEIBA and an investigational material) were studied using both the Hyland method for Factor VIII correctional units and the Immuno method for FEIBA units. Both methods were performed as done by the manufacturers using standards and reagents supplied by each company.

Preliminary results indicate that all three regular PCC (Konyne, Proplex and Prothromplex) have similar levels of Factor VIII correctional activity (7-9 U/ml) while greater activity was found in the activated products (Autoplex - 20 U/ml, FEIBA-15 U/ml, investigational product - 19 U/ml). Using the FEIBA assay, it was not possible to measure activity in the regular products since the results were non-parallel. The activated product revealed the following in the FEIBA assay:

Autoplex	- 28-40 U/ml
FEIBA	- 15-17 U/ml
Investigational product	- 25 U/ml

It is of interest that these results are consistent with our clinical experience using these products.

Until a specific assay is available for quantitating the active principle by which these materials promote haemostasis in patients with inhibitors, it would appear that the Factor VIII correctional assay and FEIBA assay will be useful for comparing the potency of products in vitro and as a guide to dosage for treatment of patients.

REFERENCES

1. Fekete, L.F., Holst, S.L., Pecetoom, F. and DeVeber, L.L. (1962). "Auto"-Factor IX concentrate: A new therapeutic approach to the treatment of haemophilia A patients with inhibitors. Presented at the Fourteenth International Congress of Haematology, Sao Paulo, Brazil, Abstr. 295

2. Kurczynski, F.M. and Penner, J. (1974). Activated prothrombin concentrate for patients with factor VIII inhibitors. N. Engl. J. Med., 291, 164

3. Abildgaard, C.F., Britton, M. and Harrison, J. (1976). Prothrombin complex concentrate (Konyne) in the treatment of haemophilic patients with factor VIII inhibitors. J. Pediatr., 88, 200

4. Sultan, U., Brouet, J.C. and Debre, P. (1974). Treatment of inhibitors to factor VIII with activated prothrombin concentrate. N. Engl. J. Med., 29, 1087

5. Goodnight, S.H., Common, H.H. and Lovrien, E.W. (1976). Factor VIII inhibitor following surgery for epidural haemorrhage in haemophilia: Successful therapy with a concentrate containing factor II, VII, IX, and X. J. Pediatr., 88, 356

6. Lowe, G.D.O., Harvie, A., Forbes, C.D. and Prentice, C.R.M. (1976). Successful treatment with prothrombin complex concentrate of postoperative bleeding in a haemophiliac with a factor VIII inhibitor. Br. J. Med., 2, 1110

7. Sonoda, T., Solomon, A., Krauss, S., Cruz, P., Jones, F.S. and Levin, J. (1976). Use of prothrombin complex concentrates in the treatment of a haemophilia patient with an inhibitor to factor VIII. Blood, 47. 983

8.   Kelly, P. and Penner, J.A. (1976). Antihaemophilic factor inhibitors. Management with prothrombin complex concentrates. J. Am. Med. Assoc., 236, 2061

9.   Rosen, R., Mikel, T. and Corrigan, J.J. (1977). Acquired circulating anticoagulant in classical haemophilia: Treatment with prothrombin concentrate. Ariz. Med., 34, 340

10. Blatt, P.M., White, G.C., McMillan, C.W. and Roberts, H.R. (1977). Treatment of anti-factor VIII antibodies. Thromb. Haemost., 38, 515

11. Buchanan, G.R. and Kevy, S.W. (1978). Use of prothrombin complex concentrates in haemophiliacs with inhibitors: Clinical and laboratory studies. Pediatrics, 65, 767

12. Yolken, R.H. and Hilgartner, M.W. (1978). Prothrombin complex concentrates. Use in treatment of haemophiliacs with factor VIII inhibitors. Am. J. Dis. Child., 132, 291

13. Manucci, P., Federici, F., Vigano, S. and Cattaneo, M. (1979). Multiple dental extractions with a new prothrombin complex concentrate in two patients with factor VIII inhibitors. Thromb. Res., 15, 359

14. Lusher, J.M., Shapiro, S.S., Palascak, J.E., Rao, A.J., Levine, P.H., Blatt, P.M. and the Hemophilia Study Group (1980). Efficacy of prothrombin-complex concentrates in haemophiliacs with antibodies to factor VIII. A Multicentre therapeutic trial. N. Engl. J. Med., 303, 421

15. Abildgaard, C.F., Penner, J.A. and Watson-Williams, E.J. (1980). Anti-Inhibitor coagulant complex (Autoplex) for treatment of factor VIII inhibitors in haemophilia. Blood (In Press)

16. Hoots, W.K., Snyder, M.S. and McMillan, C.S. (1980). Effects of activated prothrombin complex concentrates (APCC) for craniospinal haemorrhage in classic haemophiliacs with factor VIII inhibitors. Pediatr. Res., 14, 535

17. Silverstein, A. (1960). Intracranial bleeding in haemophilia. Arch Neurol., 3, 141

Discussion

<u>Prof. Stewart</u>:   The units that were used - were they your activated units? You used so many units per kilogram, 50 units/kg or 100 units/kg to treat the patients. Which units were used?

<u>Prof. Abildgaard</u>: We were using these units - the units with which they labelled the material.

<u>Prof. Stewart</u>:   But in FEIBA you got only about half the activity of the label.

<u>Prof. Abildgaard</u>: With the FEIBA we have used it according to the label. It has just been this one <u>in vitro</u> study.

<u>Dr. Stevens</u>:   Has anyone seen any anamnestic response or a rise in inhibitor titre following Autoplex?

<u>Prof. Abildgaard</u>: We have not, and as far as I know there has been none seen in the accumulated investigational period, with Autoplex. With FEIBA we have, I think, had similar experiences. In a small number of patients studied we have seen a few with anamnestic responses.

<u>Dr. Savidge</u>:   Is there any special protocol for dealing with allergic reactions?

<u>Prof. Abildgaard</u>: We have not had problems so far in our experience.

13

Immune complex disease in haemophilia

M. W. Hilgartner

The clinical manifestations of haemophilia have been significantly altered in the past 12 years through improved medical care with early transfusion for bleeding episodes and availability of lyophilized clotting factor. However, 10-15% of patients with severe deficiencies of Factor VIII and IX continue to have progressive joint disease despite adequate treatment for bleeding episodes. We have confirmed this observation of Levine[1] in an adult population and have been particularly concerned about a group of children transfused since infancy soon after onset of bleeding who now have grade III arthropathy at 5 years of age. An immune aetiology of this progressive arthropathy has been postulated as an explanation of this phenomenon. A group from the St. Mary's Hospital in London and another in L.A. Childrens' Hospital have found circulating immune complexes in approximately 30-50% of sera tested but with little, if any, correlation to clinical disease. Both noted complexes in patients with elevated liver enzymes and inhibitors and one found inhibitor activity in the complex. The development of sensitive tests for the presence of immune complexes allowed an investigation of the patients seen at our Regional Haemophilia Centre for the presence of soluble circulating immune complexes and a correlation for immune complex disease.

The sera from 73 randomly selected patients seen for primary care at The New York Hospital Hemophilia Clinic were studied for the presence of soluble immune complexes; 64 patients had severe Factor VIII deficiency of < 1%; 4 had severe Factor IX deficiency of < 1%, and 2 had severe von Willebrand's disease with < 10% of Factor VIII activity. 12 of the Factor VIII deficient patients had an inhibitor to Factor VIII.

The immune complexes were assayed by two different methods -the Raji cell method developed by Theofilopoulous, Wilson and Dixon[4] and a

143

staphylococcal binding assay developed by McDougal, Redecha, Inman and Christian[5] in our Instituation. The Raji cell is a human lymphoblastoid cell line derived from Burkitt's lymphoma with B cell characteristics. These cells lack membrane-bound immunoglobulin but have receptors for IgG, Fc, C3b, C3d and other complement proteins. Aggregated human gammaglobulin (AHG) and 7S IgG binds avidly to the complement receptors and less well to receptors for the Fc fragment. The assay is based on the ability of the Raji cells to bind human IgG much more efficiently when it is complexed with an antigen or when it is aggregated and has fixed complement than when it is in the monomeric form. The method is relatively simple; the Raji cells are incubated with the patient's serum. If complexes are present and contain complement they will bind to the complement receptors. The cells are then reacted with excess ^{125}I-rabbit anti-human IgG and the radioactivity in the spun pellet is compared to a standard curve of radioactive antibody uptake by the cells. The sensitivity of the method is 6 µg/ml. The normal range with this method as determined by Theofilopoulous et al. is < 16 µg/ml.

The staphylococcal binding assay (SBA) uses the formalin fixed Cowan I strain of Staph. aureus to bind aggregated IgG preferentially over monomeric IgG at the Fc binding site. The assay is relatively unaffected by factors such as heparin, complement, native antibodies and immunoglobulin concentrations, but is affected by the presence of rheumatoid factor. It is based on the ability of Staph. aureus to bind solubilised aggregated IgG with subsequent detection with ^{125}I-labelled rabbit antihuman IgG. Monomeric IgG is eliminated by precipitation with 5% polyethylene glycol. The immune complex in the sera is then expressed in aggregated-IgG equivalents (µg/ml) from a known standard curve, (the normal range is > 10 µg/ml). The sensitivity of the method appears to be 20% better than the CIQ binding and the Raji cell, both complement dependent assays for the complexes in rheumatoid arthritis and SLE. Both methods detect immune complexes at equivalence and in antigen excess. The advantage of the SBA over the Raji lies in its use as a tool to isolate immune complex material. Conditions can be manipulated to elute the complexes from the Staph. aureus with thiocyanate that would lyse the Raji cell.

The results in the haemophilia patients are shown in Tables 1 and 2. We chose to use the sera from multiply-transfused thalassaemics rather than normal sera for comparison and they are labelled "controls" in these tables. For patients and controls the results ranged from 0 to 2400 µg/ml by Raji assay; those in the normal group have $<$ 16 µg/ml of soluble immune complexes in their serum; the positive group 16 – 2400 µg/ml; 23, or 50% of the haemophiliacs, had elevated immune complexes in their serum. The difference between the haemophiliac group and the controls was found to be highly significant by the chi square test with $p < 0.005$.

For the SBA assay 10% of the haemophiliacs and 25% of the controls have normal values while 90% of haemophiliacs are positive. The p value is significant to < 0.01 level.

Table 1   Immune complex levels in haemophiliacs and multiply-transfused controls (Raji method)

	Controls	Haemophiliacs
Number tested	28	46
Normal (<16 µg/ml)	20 (71%)	23 (50%)
Elevated (>16 µg/ml)	8 (29%)	23 (50%)

chi^2 = 4.5851 $p < 0.05$

The abnormal groups were examined separately for possible correlates. Patient age, factor deficiency, brand of lyophilized concentrate used and number of units infused per year were examined and could not be correlated with immune complex levels.

The ages of the haemophiliacs are equally distributed in each group: 5-45 years in all groups, whereas the thalassaemics are 16-31 years of age, with the highest levels occurring in the oldest patients who have severe heart and liver dysfunction.

Although the majority of the patients had Factor VIII deficiency, the 4 Factor IX deficient patients were equally distributed with 2 in the normal range and 2 with elevated complex levels by Raji, and elevated by SBA.

Table 2   Immune complex levels in haemophiliacs and multiply-transfused controls (SBA method)

	Controls		Haemophiliacs	
Number tested	12		73	
Normal (<10 μg/ml)	3	(25%)	7	(10%)
Elevated (>10 μg/ml)	9	(75%)	66	(90%)

chi^2 = 7.548 p < 0.01

The concentrates were not limited to one manufacturer since we have a monthly rotational buying system for all products and immune complex levels were not found in the 6 Factor VIII and 2 Factor IX products tested by Raji cell. The amount of replacement product was very similar in all groups with 1208–1350 units/kg infused per patient per year. The lower infusion amount was used by those with normal levels of complexes but is not significantly different from those with elevated complex levels.

The complex levels are variable in any one patient using both techniques. 5 patients have had high levels of complexes present at one testing and normal levels at another; 3 patients have had consistently elevated levels on two or more testings and one patient has had two high levels and one normal. These values have not been correlated with exact time of infusion since all samples were drawn at the time of clinic visit at least 72 hours after an infusion. However, it is assumed that the complexes are produced in a state of antigen excess as occurs following a transfusion.

Figure 1 illustrates the formation of the immune complexes following a transfusion of Factor VIII concentrate. The three points to be noted are: (1) the rise of Factor VIII clotting activity and its fall off with a $t_\frac{1}{2}$ of 5½ hours, (2) the rise in plasma level of Factor VIII antigen at the usual time of 1 hour after infusion with its rapid fall off, much more rapid than expected, to the patient's own baseline of around 300 μg/100 ml and, finally, (3) the appearance of the immune complexes and their clearing in

6-7 hours to below the patient's baseline value. Multiple baseline samples from this patient have ranged from 590 to 1600 with a mean of 960 µg/ml by Raji cell.

The complexes were isolated by SBA from this patient (R.B.) and from a patient (J.S.) with a Factor VIII inhibitor of 60 BU (Bethesda units) and characterised on a sucrose gradient. Figure 2 is the sucrose gradient of the complex from the patient R.B. whose survival data was shown in Figure 1. The graph from J.S. is similar. The one peak suggests a homogeneous complex shifted towards the heavy 7S globulins which, on Ouchterlony plates, was found to contain only IgG.

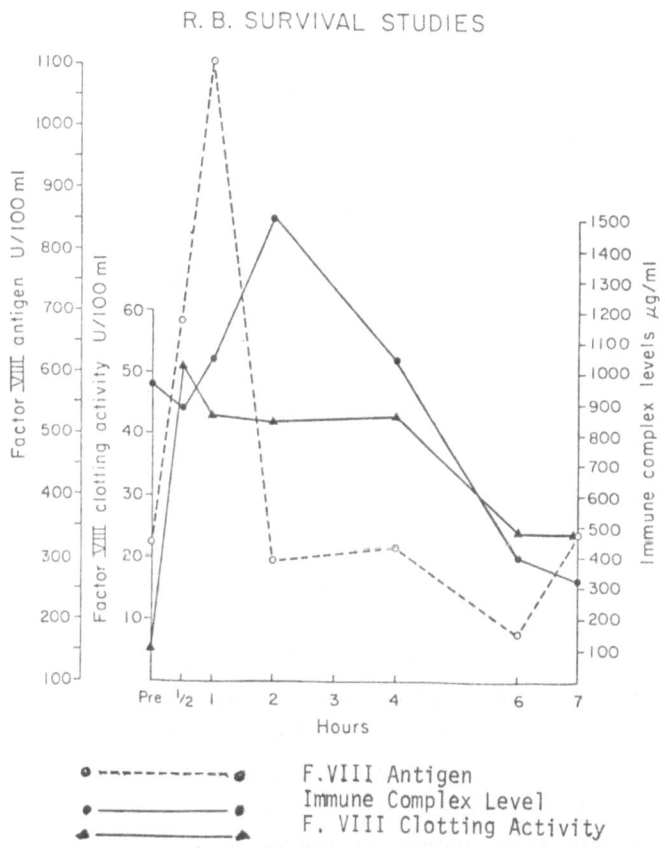

Figure 1   Formation of immune complexes following a transfusion of Factor VIII concentrate

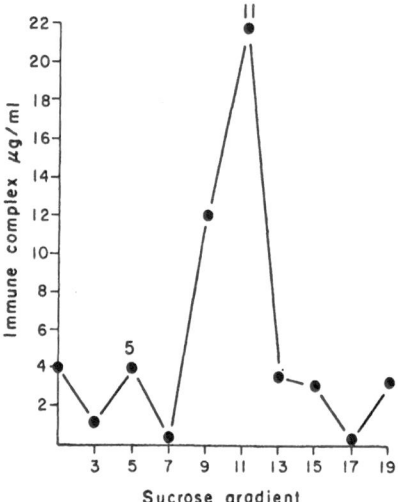

Figure 2   Sucrose gradient of immune complex isolated from patient R.B.

The complexes were isolated and assayed for Factor VIII coagulant antigen by radioimmunoassay. Small amounts of Factor VIII antigen were found; < 0.6 U/100 ml are present in R.B.'s complex and < 0.3 U/100 ml in the complex of J.S. who had the Factor VIII inhibitor. Small amounts of Factor VIII antigen were remaining in the serum wtih 7.8 U/100 ml in R.B. and 1.7 U/100 ml in J.S. The data suggests Factor VIII may be present in this complex but needs to be pursued further.

The clinical significance of these complexes was considered and the presence of immune complex disease sought. Data collected over the preceeding 5 years relating to liver disease, joint disease and renal disease (complex disease in other settings) were tabulated and correlated with the presence of the immune complexes in haemophilia. These parameters of known disease in the haemophiliac were considered as complications of the therapy or complications of the disease itself. The patients were scored as positive or negative for each of these parameters and the results are shown in Table 3. Liver disease was defined as present if one of the transaminases was twice normal on two or more testings and hepatitis B surface antibody was present.

Hepatitis B exposure was present in almost all the patients tested; 41 and 64 respectively were hepatitis B antibody positive. The remaining patients are hepatitis antigen positive and are carriers. There is no correlation of patients with positive liver disease and elevated complexes by either method.

Table 3   Clinical features.   Factor VIII inhibitor status vs. immune complex levels

	RAJI		SBA	
	Number studied*	Inhibitor >1 BU	Number studied*	Inhibitor >1 BU
Normal	21	3 (14%)	6	1 (17%)
Elevated	21	8 (38%)**	58	11 (19%)

*   Factor IX deficient patients omitted.

**   Significantly different from normal group,
      p < 0.05

Severe chronic synovitis was considered present if at least two joints were involved with synovial hypertrophy and had the changes of chronic arthropathy. With chronic synovitis there is a significant increase among those with elevated complexes, significant to p < 0.05 by Raji cell only.

Haemophilic renal disease was defined as present if the patient had more than one episode of gross haematuria. Although the numbers are small, the increase in renal disease with haematuria was significant to p < 0.05 by both methods. Thus, the presence of elevated serum immune complexes seems to correlate well with the clinical manifestations of joint disease and renal disease in the haemophilia population and is highly suggestive of immune complex disease. A single joint fluid was tested for complexes in the presence of added complement and found positive. The chronic arthropathy may indeed be a manifestation of an immune response with the deposition of immune complexes in the synovium as part of the destructive process.

Table 4   Clinical features vs. immune complex levels

| IC level | Severe chronic synovitis | | Haematuria | |
	Raji	SBA	Raji	SBA
Normal	13 (57%)	6 (86%)	2 (9%)	0
Elevated	19 (83%)*	48 (73%)	10 (43%)*	18 (27%)*

* significantly different from normal group, $p < 0.05$

The correlation of Factor VIII inhibitor status and the presence of immune complexes is extremely significant – $p < 0.05$ with the Raji cell data, but was not present in the SBA.

Table 5   Clinical features.   Factor VIII inhibitor status vs. immune complex levels

| | RAJI | | SBA | |
	Number studied*	Inhibitor >1 BU	Number studied*	Inhibitor >1 BU
Normal	21	3 (14%)	6	1 (17%)
Elevated	21	8 (38%)**	58	11 (19%)

*   Factor IX deficient patients omitted.

**   Significantly different from normal group,
      $p < 0.05$

Immune complex disease has been studied by Dixon in rabbits given daily i.p. injections of antigens. Those who were good responders and developed antibodies, did not develop chronic immune complex lesions, presumably because the complexes formed after each injection were cleared rapidly. Those animals which were not good responders and failed to produce antibodies, <u>did not</u> develop lesions. However, those animals with moderate antibody response had circulating complexes <u>and developed the lesions of chronic immune complex disease.</u>

Using the animal model, we postulated a similar process may be present in the haemophiliacs who have already produced one antibody and have an inhibitor to Factor VIII activity. In Table 6 the presence of the immune complex is correlated with the presence of Factor VIII inhibitors. Of the 11 patients who have inhibitors, 8 have complexes present by Raji. Of the group with intermediate amount of complexes present (16500 µg/ml - the moderate antibody response), 5 (50%) have inhibitors. This number is significantly different from the group with normal levels (low responders) and the group with high levels (> 500 µg/ml - the good responders with little disease).   In addition, the inhibitor titres tend to be higher in the normal group av. 110 BU, while the intermediate group av. 21 BU, and the high titre complex group have av. 6.2 BU inhibitor titre. The inhibitor titres tend to be inverse to the immune complexes.

Table 6   Immune complex and Factor VIII inhibitors

IC level	No. studied*	Inhibitor titre > 1 BU	
Normal	21	3	(14%)
Intermediate	10	5	(50%)**
High	11	3	(27%)

*   Factor IX deficient patients omitted.
**   Significantly different from normal group, $p < 0.005$.

The example of complex formation in the high responder group shown in Figures 1 and 2 may substantiate this theory. The complex levels were certainly cleared, but only to the baseline level of 300 µg/ml which is still well above normal. The slow clearing of this level of complexes might well have been accomplished with deposition in the tissues, particularly the synovium with the development of severe arthropathy. The patient has had sufficient arthropathy to require bilateral knee arthroplasties.

The differences between the two test results need to be discussed. They might be due to different patients in each group, since simultaneous samples were not used. The characteristics of each group were tabulated and are shown in Table 7.

One can readily appreciate that the groups are amazingly similar: 20-26% have an inhibitor to Factor VIII; 88-89% are positive for hepatitis surface antigen; 52-54% have evidence of liver disease, with one of the enzymes SGOT/SGPT twice normal on two or more testings; 70-74% have synovial hypertrophy and haematuria was present on more than one occasion in 25-26%.

Table 7   Characterisation of test groups

	Raji study	SBA study
Inhibitor present	26%	20%
HB$_s$Ab+	89%	88%
SGOT/SGPT ↑	54%	52%
Synovitis present	70%	74%
Haematuria present	26%	25%

If the characteristics of the patients are so strikingly similar it may well be asked why there appears to be a greater percentage of immune complexes detected by the SBA assay rather than the Raji assay, in both the controls and the study group. 90% of the patients are positive by SBA while 50% are positive by Raji. The Raji cell detects only those complexes aggregated with complement while the SBA detects a far wider group of non-specific complexes; or perhaps the SBA is picking up a larger group of specific complexes with multiple antigenic stimuli. Only when we have isolated more complexes for identification can we answer that question.

SUMMARY

1.   Circulating immune complexes are present in the serum of 50% of the

haemophiliacs tested by Raji cell and in 90% of those tested by SBA.

2. These complexes cannot be correlated with age, clotting factors deficiency or the type and amount of replacement therapy given.

3. The immune complexes are gammaglobulins, 1gG in type and appear homogeneous in nature.

4. The complexes are formed rapidly, within 2 hours, in the presence of Factor VIII antigen excess given by concentrate and cleared within 6 hours to the patient's baseline level.

5. The aetiology of the complex is unknown and is probably heterogenous in nature, and may be due to multiple transfused antigens of which Factor VIII appears to be one such antigen. In some patients an immune response to a foreign or altered Factor VIII may play a role. Work in progress suggests complexes are also found in the haemophiliacs with the hepatitis B surface antigen.

6. A significant correlation exists between the presence of immune complexes and chronic synovitis and haematuria, suggesting the presence of immune complex disease, very similar to that found in rheumatoid arthritis, systemic lupus, and the hepatitis polyarthritis syndrome.

7. A significant number of patients with an inhibitor to Factor VIII clotting activity have elevated immune complexes present by the Raji method.

8. Investigations of additional antigens responsible for the immune response are on-going.

9. Determinations of tissue deposition of the immune complexes remain to be done.

REFERENCES

1. Levine, P.H. (1974). Efficacy of self-therapy in hemophilia. A study of 72 patients with haemophilia A and B. N. Engl. J. Med., 291, 1381

2. Kazachkine, M., Mowbray, J.F., Burton, E.J. and Sultan, Y. (1978). Circulating immune complexes in haemophilia. Abstract. Clin. Res. p. 350 A

3. Gomperts, E.D., Berg, D., Sakai, R.S. and Jordan, S.C. (1980). Circulating immune complexes (CICS) in haemophilia before and after factor infusion. Abstract. Proceeds 18th Cong. of Int. Soc. Hem. p.190

4. Theofilopoulus, A.N., Wilson, C.B. and Dixon, F.S. (1976). The Raji cell radioimmune assay for detecting immune complexes in human sera. J. Clin. Invest., 57, 569

5. McDougal, J.S., Redecha, P.B., Inman, R.D. and Christian, C.L. (1979). Binding of IgG aggregates and immune complexes in human sera to Staphylococci containing protein A. Am. J. Clin. Invest., 63, 627

Discussion

Dr. Preston: Can we be certain that there are no complexes in the therapeutic material which you are giving.

Prof. Hilgartner: We have tested 6 of the concentrates that we have used. We have done 4 Factor VIII and 2 of the Factor IX preparations and we have not found complexes present in those particular lots.

Dr. Tuddenham: We reported in 1979 a haemophilic with high titre of inhibitor who consistently gets nephrotic syndrome after infusion with Factor VIII. There are reports in the literature on 2 similar described cases who had similar problems associated with transfusion. Both those previously described cases and our own patient had a potent GM antibody. Have you looked at GM antibodies?

Prof. Hilgartner: No. That we have not done.

Dr. Giddings: Is the Factor VIII inhibitor antigen reaction interpreted as being complement-dependent?

Prof. Hilgartner: It seems to be, at least in the 2 methods that we have used. That does not seem to be the conclusion in one of the other authors I know who had looked at this in the literature.

Dr. Prentice: I know that Prof. Hilgartner is worried about linking the immune complex deposition of haematuria. We looked at quite a lot of patients with haematuria, and they did not have the presence of white cells or granular casts which we associate with immune complex disease. We concluded that these were small leaking vessels with red cell loss. Has any evidence been found of immune complex damage in the kidneys of these patients over and above pure haematuria?

Dr. Hilgartner: No, we have not found any, and the only ones that I know of are 2 patients who have developed very severe renal disease and one has required a transplant.

Dr. Prentice: I agree that some have been reported as developing it, but in your series there did not seem to be a big tie up between haematuria and immune complexes.

Prof. Hilgartner: No.

Dr. Wensley: Have you found that patients with mild haemophilia who develop antibodies are more likely to have immune complexes?

Prof. Hilgartner: For some strange reason, we had very few patients with mild disease in our clinic. In fact, we have only 3. That probably means that we have a particularly select group who come to us. So I cannot answer that question, because we just do not have any with mild disease.

Prof. Bloom: In the operated patients - one synovectomy patient was mentioned - were any histological changes seen which could be consistent with immune complex formation?

Prof. Hilgartner: That particular patient had both knees replaced and at the time they were replaced he had no synovium left that could be looked at. We do have several other people who are sending samples and we hope we can do just that.

Dr. Rizza: I wanted to ask if there was any evidence that synovitis was less before 1965 when concentrate therapy started?

Prof. Hilgartner: I do not think it was less. It was probably greater. That was one of the reasons for comparing the amount of product that was used. We do not think that it is necessarily related to the amount of product, but that it probably has a patient-related response - an individual patient response. We only have this in about 10–15 per cent of the patients.

Prof. Bloom: Can the release of blood into the tissues, even in the absence of any form of treatment, reveal new antigens which can then stimulate the formation of antibodies and lead to possible changes?

Prof. Hilgartner: That was one of the theories we were going to go on several years ago, and thought that perhaps some of the red cell antigens themselves might be changed within the synovial tissue but we had not been able to progress with it.

Factor VIII – Structure, Function and Genetics

14 Factor VIII – structure and function

L. Hoyer

The importance of Factor VIII in haemostasis and blood coagulation is obvious from the clinical problems in the Factor VIII deficiency diseases, classic haemophilia and von Willebrand's disease. During the past decade there has been intense research interest in these diseases, the two most common hereditary bleeding disorders, and in the properties of Factor VIII. These studies have provided an evolving understanding of Factor VIII structure and function.

The concept that Factor VIII has two distinct biological functions -- coagulant activity and a role in primary haemostasis -- has evolved from the recognition of a dual defect in von Willebrand's disease and from recent biochemical and immunological studies (Table 1).

Table 1   The components of the Factor VIII complex

Factor VIII procoagulant activity (VIII:C)
    Antihaemophilic factor activity. The procoagulant property of normal plasma that is measured by standard Factor VIII coagulation assays.

Factor VIII procoagulant antigen (VIII:CAg)
    Antigenic determinants closely associated with VIII:C. Measured with human antibodies.

Factor VIII-related protein (VIIIR)
    The large polymeric protein that is necessary for normal platelet adhesion and bleeding time in vivo and is measured in vitro by VIIIR:Ag and ristocetin cofactor assays. Also designated von Willebrand factor since it is reduced in that disease.

Factor VIII-related antigen (VIIIR:Ag)

Antigenic determinants on VIIIR that are detected by heterologous antibodies.

Ristocetin cofactor (VIIIR:RC)

The property of VIIIR in normal plasma that supports ristocetin-induced agglutination of washed normal platelets.

It is now generally recognised that plasma Factor VIII is a complex of two components that have distinct functions, biochemical properties, genetic control and antigenic determinants (Figure 1). One component of the Factor VIII complex has antihaemophilic factor procoagulant activity (VIII:C) and can be identified by human antibodies (as VIII:CAg). The other, larger component, Factor VIII related protein (VIIIR), comprises the majority of the protein mass, interacts with platelets in a way that promotes primary haemostasis, and forms immunoprecipitates with heterologous antisera.

Several kinds of data have led to the differentiation of the two proteins:

1. VIII:C and VIIIR are controlled by different genes: VIII:C is an X chromosome product and VIIIR is controlled by an autosomal gene.

2. The proteins are separable in buffers of high ionic strength (1 mol/l NaCl or 0.24 mol/l $CaCl_2$) [1-4].

3. The plasma concentrations vary independently under certain conditions, the best known being the post-transfusion period in patients with von Willebrand's disease [5].

4. The two proteins have different antigenic determinants: VIII:C is inactivated by human antibodies; ristocetin cofactor activity is inhibited by rabbit antisera. There is little or no cross-reactivity, and each can be measured by an immunoassay that is independent of the other protein [6,7].

5.   VIII:C retains full activity in the virtual absence of VIIIR[8] (i.e. an VIII:C/VIIIR:Ag ratio of 12,600:1[8] as does VIIIR:RC in the absence of detectable VIII:C[9].

The two components of the Factor VIII complex do interact, however. Their concentrations vary together under most normal, stressful and pathological situations, and standard purification methods separate the intact (two component) Factor VIII complex from other plasma proteins.

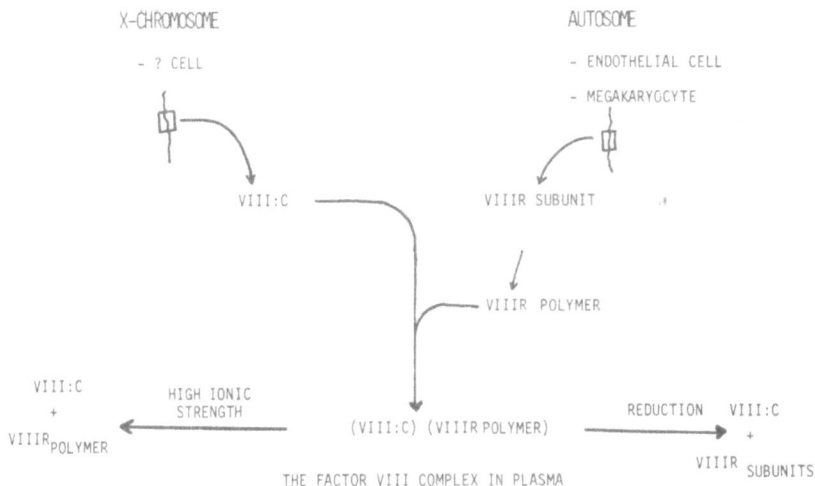

Figure 1   The Factor VIII complex. This interpretation indicates the interaction of the two components and their genetic control. The effects of high ionic strength and reduction are noted

FACTOR VIII PROCOAGULANT PROTEIN: ANTIHAEMOPHILIC FACTOR

Biochemical Properties

At the present time, there is little published information about the biochemical properties of VIII:C, per se. With few exceptions, studies of VIII:C function have been carried out with the intact Factor VIII complex and it is only recently that VIII:C has been studied after separation from VIIIR and other plasma proteins[8].

The molecular weight of human VIII:C separated from VIIIR is ca. 285,000[10]. This value has been obtained by a combination of Sephadex G-200 gel filtration measurements (with calculation of Stokes' radius) and sucrose density gradient centrifugation (8.2S). These properties of unactivated VIII:C are very similar to those recently obtained for Factor V by Nesheim and co-workers[11].

Immunological Properties

Human anti-VIII:C, obtained from multitransfused haemophilic patients that develop inhibitors and from rare individuals who form autoantibodies that inactivate VIII:C, does not form detectable immunoprecipitates with VIII:C or with the Factor VIII complex. Nevertheless, these sera can be used to detect VIII:C antigenic determinants by sensitive immunoradiometric assays[7,12].

In general, there is excellent correlation between the Factor VIII procoagulant activity and the VIII:CAg content in normal human plasma (Figure 2). Serum VIII:CAg values are 60-80% of those in the corresponding plasma sample.

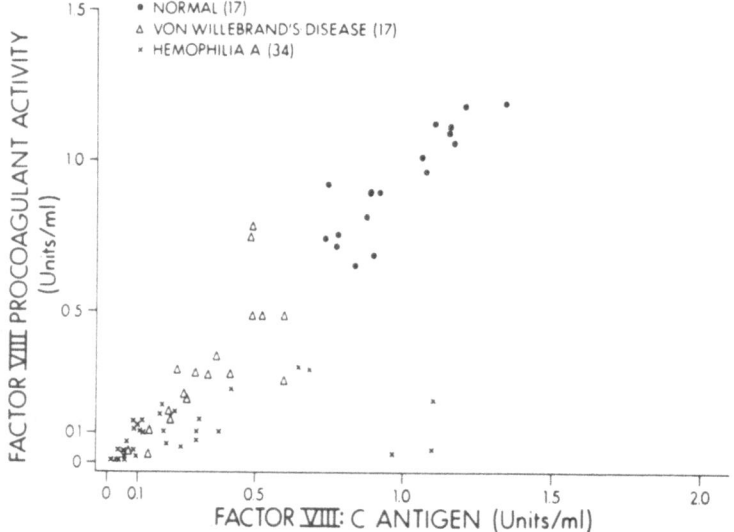

Figure 2   The relationship of VIII:C procoagulant activity and VIII:CAg. Modified from Lazarchick and Hoyer[7]

Function

VIII:C accelerates blood coagulation by its effect on the enzymatic activation of factor X by Factor IX_a in the presence of phospholipid and calcium. VIII:C serves as a cofactor in this reaction; it does not have any intrinsic capacity to activate Factor X[13].

The form in which VIII:C participates in this reaction is somewhat less certain. Early studies established that VIII:C activity is enhanced when plasma or Factor VIII concentrates are incubated with dilute thrombin. They suggested in fact, that thrombin activation is essential for VIII:C activity.

It is presumed that thrombin activates VIII:C by proteolysis, and this effect has been demonstrated in recent studies that have identified a thrombin-induced shift in human VIII:C gel filtration properties (Figure 3). VIII:C inactivation by higher concentrations of thrombin -- or more prolonged exposure to the enzyme -- caused a further change in the elution properties of the (non-functional) protein measured by VIII:CAg assays (Figure 3C).

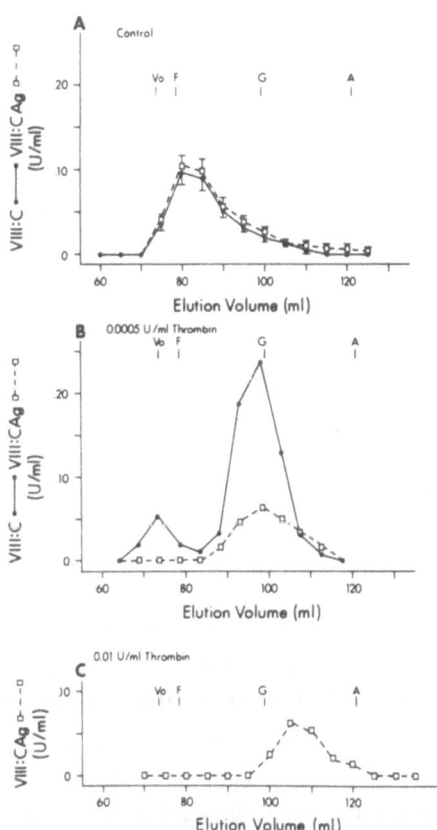

Figure 3   The Sephadex G-200 gel filtration properties of purified VIII:C. The void volume (V_o) is indicated as are the elution properties Modified from Hoyer and Trabold[10]

of IgG (G), fibrinogen (F) and albumin (A).

A. VIII:C free of detectable VIIIR.

B. VIIIR:C incubated with 5×10^{-4} U/ml human thrombin for 4 hours at 37 °C.

C. VIII:C incubated with 10^{-2} U/ml human thrombin for 4 hours at 37 °C.

FACTOR VIII-RELATED PROTEIN: VON WILLEBRAND FACTOR

Biochemical Properties

As the bulk of the Factor VIII complex is made up of VIIIR, data obtained for the intact Factor VIII complex are actually VIIIR properties.

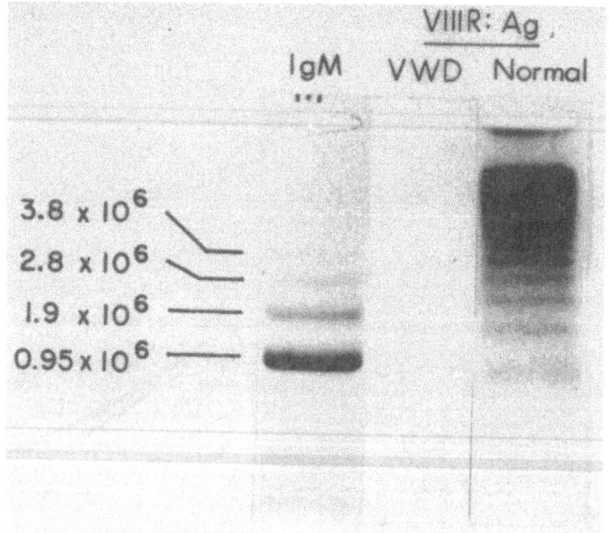

Figure 4   The polymer pattern of human VIIIR analysed by SDS-agarose electrophoresis. The migration of IgM and IgM polymers is indicated on the left and their molecular weights are noted. The proteins of the two other samples were separated by SDS-agarose electrophoresis and the VIIIR:Ag identified by autoradiography after incubation with iodine-125 labelled rabbit anti-VIIIR:Ag. There is no detectable VIIIR:Ag in the plasma from a patient with severe von Willebrand's disease.
Modified from Hoyer and Shainoff [16]

Purified VIIIR protein is very large by all criteria, and a molecular weight of 1.12×10^6 has been obtained in sedimentation equilibrum studies carried out in 6 mol/l guanidine[14]. Agarose gel filtration separations also indicate a molecular weight greater than one million[1-3]. When reduced, VIIIR is composed of homogeneous subunits that have a molecular weight of 195,000–230,000[9,14,15]. Small forms are not detectable in normal human plasma, however, and VIIIR is composed of a population of large multimers with molecular weights between 0.85×10^6 and approximately 12×10^6 (Figure 4). The very large polymers are detected in fresh normal plasma and, presumably, are present in vivo. They do not reflect aggregation induced by calcium chelation, freezing or purification[16].

The normal plasma concentration of VIIIR, estimated from the specific activity of highly purified protein, is between 5–10 µg/ml.

Immunological Properties

After appropriate absorptions, rabbit antisera to human factor VIII form a single immunoprecipitation line when tested with normal human plasma[17]. A number of different assays have been used to detect and quantify this Factor VIII-related antigen. Laurell electroimmunoassay, counter immuno electrophoresis, and radioimmunoassay all give similar results[5,6,17].

In general, there is an excellent correlation between VIII:C activity and VIIIR:Ag in normal human plasmas[6,17]. Parallel increases in VIII:C and VIIIR:Ag have been noted in plasmas from patients with a wide range of non-haematological diseases and from normal individuals subjected to physiological stimuli[5].

Von Willebrand Factor Activity

Factor VIII-related protein has a central role in normal platelet function and the prolonged bleeding time in von Willebrand's disease is presumed to be the reduced plasma VIIIR content[5]. The two in vitro platelet assays that are abnormal in von Willebrand's disease (ristocetin-induced platelet agglutination and retention of platelets in glass bead columns) are corrected by purified normal Factor VIII[5]. Although there are exceptions, there is usually a good correlation between the prolonged bleeding time in von Willebrand's disease and reduced plasma VIIIR:Ag and ristocetin cofactor activity (VIIIR:RC)[18]. Recent in vitro studies suggest that only large VIIIR polymers bind to platelets and have ristocetin cofactor activity[19,20].

THE INTERACTION OF VIII:C and VIIIR IN THE FACTOR VIII COMPLEX

Although VIII:C and VIIIR have very distinct properties, it would be incorrect to suggest that they are simply two proteins that happen to copurify. Several observations suggest that they are associated in a non-covalent complex, but there is only indirect evidence for a high-affinity interaction in plasma. For example, the concentrations of the two proteins are closely correlated in normal plasmas and in most (non-haematological) disease states[5]. In addition, rabbit anti-VIIIR coupled to agarose removes similar amounts of VIII:C and VIIIR from plasma[8]. If VIII:C and VIIIR did not interact, there would be no basis for the VIII:C loss in these experiments.

The effect of reducing agents on plasma VIII:C also suggest that there is a relatively high-affinity interaction with VIIIR. In contrast to its properties in native plasma, VIII:C in plasma exposed to low concentrations of dithiothreitol or mercaptoethanol has the characteristics of a relatively small protein on sucrose density centrifugation, agarose gel filtration, and ethanol precipitation[21]. While this change could be due to a direct effect of the reducing agent on VIII:C, the "normal" properties return when VIIIR (haemophilic plasma) is added.

THE FACTOR VIII DEFICIENCY DISEASES

Haemophilia A

Although the low Factor VIII concentration in plasma has prevented biochemical studies in classic haemophilia (haemophilia A), immunological techniques have begun to define the molecular defect. The initial studies, carried out with the heterologous antisera, identified normal VIIIR:Ag levels in haemophilia[6,17]. It is now apparent that these results do not demonstrate an intact Factor VIII complex, only normal VIIIR:Ag synthesis as one would expect from the normal bleeding time.

The antigens detected by human anti-factor VIII are more clearly related to VIII:C. Early studies, carried out by antibody neutralisation assays, demonstrated non-functional VIII:C-like material in approximately 10% of haemophilic plasmas, usually those with low (2-10%) activity[22]. These observations have been expanded as quantitative immunoradiometric assays have been developed and several different patterns have been identified in haemophilic plasmas (Figure 2).

Neither VIII:C nor VIII:CAg are detectable in most plasmas from patients with severe haemophilia. Low VIII:CAg levels -- 1-10% of normal -- are present in ca. 25% of these patients, however, even though VIII:C is <0.01 U/ml. Variable VIII:CAg levels are observed in mild and moderate haemophilia; usually there is slightly more immunoreactive material than VIII:C. In contrast, a small group of haemophilic plasmas have normal VIII:CAg even though the coagulant activity is low. These plasmas are the same ones that are identified as CRM+ by antibody neutralisation assays[7]. Thus, non-functional VIII:C-like molecules are synthesized by some haemophilic patients. The reduction of VIII:CAg in the remaining patients may reflect a defect that is so severe that antigenic reactivity is lost or there may be a diminution or absence of the VIII:C protein.

Von Willebrand's Disease

Immunological, biochemical and functional assays have also clarified our understanding of von Willebrand's disease. In this case, the haemostatic disorder is caused by genetic abnormalities of the VIIIR autosomal locus. Qualitative and quantitative VIIIR defects have been identified in this disease; the reduced VIII:C levels appear to be secondary.

In its most frequent form, von Willebrand's disease is a mild or moderate bleeding disorder characterised by reduced plasma content of all components of the Factor VIII complex and a slightly long bleeding time[5]. While VIII:C and VIII:CAg may be slightly higher than VIIIR:Ag and VIIIR:RC, the values are usually similar (Figure 2)[5,18]. In general, the bleeding time prolongation corresponds to the severity of the VIIIR reduction and there is a reduced concentration of both large and small VIIIR polymers[20].

Severe von Willebrand's disease is a very different, and rare,

168

condition in which individuals have very low levels of all Factor VIII properties, a markedly prolonged bleeding time, and a major bleeding diathesis. Family studies often demonstrate that these patients are homozygous offspring of parents with mild, or asymptomatic, von Willebrand's disease.

It is not certain why VIII:C is low in von Willebrand's disease, for these patients have the genetic capacity to form VIII:C. This potential is expressed after transfusion of normal plasma, cryoprecipitate or factor VIII concentrates[5]. Recent studies suggest that normal VIIIR protects VIII:C from inactivation[24]; it is possible that VIIIR deficiency permits VIII:C inactivation in vivo. It is also possible that VIIIR may affect VIII:C synthesis or its release into the plasma[25].

Most patients with von Willebrand's disease have similar levels of the different Factor VIII properties -- and this has been designated the "classical" pattern. There is heterogeneity, however, and non-functional VIIIR has been detected in some patients. These individuals have normal or slightly reduced VIII:C and VIIIR:Ag levels, very low VIIIR:RC activity, and a prolonged bleeding time. The VIIIR:Ag pattern is abnormal on crossed immunoelectrophoresis because there is an increased proportion of small VIIIR polymers and an absence of the largest forms[20]. Since platelet binding, VIIIR:RC activity, and bleeding time correction require large VIIIR polymers, their deficiency causes a bleeding diathesis. This variant form of von Willebrand's disease has been designated "type II" by some investigators to distinguish it from the more common "type I" pattern.

SUMMARY

Several different kinds of studies indicate that a complex of two distinct proteins is responsible for plasma Factor VIII activities. The proteins are under separate genetic control, have distinct biochemical properties, and have unique and essential physiological properties. While the nature of their interaction and the details of their biochemical structure remain to be determined, the available studies provide a reasonable interpretation of the Factor VIII deficiency diseases.

ACKNOWLEDGEMENT

Research studies described in this chapter have been supported by

research grants HL 16626 and HL 16872 from the United States Public Health
Service.

REFERENCES

1. Owen, W.G. and Wagner, R.H. (1972). Antihaemophilic factor:
Separation of an active fragment following dissociation by salts or
detergents. Thromb. Diath. Haemorrh., 27, 502–515

2. Rick, M.E. and Hoyer, L.W. (1973). Immunologic studies of
antihemophilic factor (AHF, factor VIII). V. Immunologic properties
of AHF subunits produced by salt dissociation. Blood, 42, 737–747

3. Weiss, H.J. and Hoyer, L.W. (1973). von Willebrand factor:
Dissociation from antihemophilic factor procoagulant activity. Science,
182, 1149–1151

4. Poon, M.C. and Ratnoff, O.D. (1976). Evidence that functional
subunits of antihemophilic factor (factor VIII) are linked by
non-covalent bonds. Blood, 48, No. 1, 87–94

5. Hoyer, L.W. (1976). von Willebrand's disease. Edited by
T.H. Spaet. In Progress in Hemostasis and Thrombosis, Vol 3. pp.
231–287 (New York: Grune and Stratton)

6. Hoyer, L.W. (1972). Immunologic studies of antihemophilic factor
(AHF, factor VIII). IV. Radioimmunoassay of AHF antigen. J. Lab.
Clin. Med., 80, 822–833

7. Lazarchick, J. and Hoyer, L.W. (1978). Immunoradiometric
measurement of the factor VIII procoagulant antigen. J. Clin.
Invest., 62, 1048–1052

8. Tuddenham, E.G.D., Trabold, N.C., Collins, J.A. et al. (1979).
The properties of factor VIII coagulant activity prepared by
immuno-adsorbent chromatography. J. Lab. Clin Med., 93, 1, 40–53

9. Olson, J.D., Brockway, W.J., Fass, D.N. et al. (1977). Purification
of porcine and human ristocetin–Willebrand factor. J. Lab. Clin.
Med., 89, 1278–1294

10. Hoyer, L.W. and Trabold, N.C. (1981). The effect of thrombin on human factor VIII. Cleavage of the factor VIII procoagulant protein during activation. (In press)

11. Nesheim, M.E., Myrmel, K.H., Hibbard, L. and Mann K.G. (1979). Isolation and characterisation of single chain bovine factor V. J. Biol. Chem., 254, 508-517

12. Peake, I.R., Bloom, A.L., Giddings, J.C. et al. (1979). An immunoradiometric assay for procoagulant factor VIII antigen: Results in haemophilia, von Willebrand's disease and fetal plasma and serum. Br. J. Haematol., 42, 269-281

13. Hultin, M.B. and Nemerson, Y. (1978). Activation of factor X by factors IX_a and VIII; a specific assay for factor IX_a in the presence of thrombin-activated factor VIII. Blood, 52, 928-940

14. Legaz, M.E., Schmer, G., Counts, R.B. et al (1973). Isolation and characterisation of human factor VIII (antihemophilic factor). J. Biol. Chem., 248, 3946-3955

15. Counts, R.B., Paskell, S.L. and Elgee, S.K. (1978). Disulfide bonds and the quaternary structure of factor VIII/von Willebrand factor J. Clin. Invest., 62, 702-708

16. Hoyer, L.W. and Shainoff, J. (1980). Factor VIII-related protein is a high molecular weight multimeric protein in normal human plasma. Blood, 55, 1056-1059

17. Zimmerman, T.S., Ratnoff, O.D. and Powell, A.E. (1971). Immunologic differentiation of classic hemophilia (factor VIII deficiency) and von Willebrand's disease, with observations on combined deficiencies of antihaemophilic factor and proaccelerin (factor V) and an acquired circulating anticoagulant against antihemophilic factor. J. Clin. Invest., 50, 244-254

18. Weiss, H.J., Hoyer, L.W., Rickles, F.R. et al. (1973). Quantitative assay of a plasma factor, deficient in von Willebrand's disease, that is necessary for platelet aggregation. Relationship to factor VIII

procoagulant activity and antigen content. J. Clin. Invest., 52, 2708-2716

19. Doucet-deBrunine, M.H.M., Sixma, J. J., Over, J. et al. (1978). Heterogeneity of human factor VIII. II. Characterisation of forms of factor VIII binding to platelets in the presence of ristocetin. J. Lab. Clin. Med., 92, 96-107

20. Ruggeri, Z.M. and Zimmerman, T.S. (1980). Variant von Willebrand's disease. J. Clin. Invest., 65, 1318-1325

21. Blomback, B., Hessel, B., Savidge, G., Wikstrom, L. and Blomback, M. (1978). The effect of reducing agents on Factor VIII and other coagulation factors. Thrombosis Res., 12, 1177-1194

22. Hoyer, L.W. and Breckenridge, R.T. (1968). Immunologic studies of antihemophilic factor (AHF, factor VIII): Cross-reacting material in a genetic variant of hemophilia A. Blood, 32, 962-971

23. Firshein, S.I., Hoyer, L.W. Lazarchick, J. et al. (1979). Prenatal diagnosis of classic hemophilia. N. Engl. J. Med., 300, 937-941

24. Weiss, H.J., Sussman, I.I. and Hoyer, L.W. (1977). Stabilisation of factor VIII in plasma by the von Willebrand factor. J. Clin. Invest., 60, 390-404

25. Owen, C.A., Jr., Bowie, E.J.W., and Fass, D.N. (1979). Generation of factor VIII coagulant activity by isolated, perfused neonatal pig livers and adult rat livers. Br. J. Haematol., 43, 307-315

Discussion

Prof. Bloom: Have you noticed any difference between the range of polymers on close examination in different individuals?

<u>Prof. Hoyer</u>:   We have just begun to do densitometry and until we are able to put quantitative numbers on it I would not be sure. But, looking at maybe 15 or 20 normals, by the eye we have not seen any differences at all. But next to each other we cannot tell which is which.

I do not think large differences will be identified, but as yet we have no quantitative data.

<u>Dr. Tuddenham</u>:   Looking at the size of the molecular weights which you got, was there much difference and can you say anything about symmetry?

<u>Prof. Hoyer</u>:   The combination of Stokes radius that we obtained by gel filtration and 8.2S ultracentrifugation suggests a very asymmetric molecule. Not quite as asymmetric as fibrinogen, but very close to it. I do not remember the numbers off hand, but that was quite striking.

<u>Prof. Bloom</u>:   Have you managed to get high-specific activity human anti CAg and stain? Do all the polymers carry CAg?

<u>Prof. Hoyer</u>:   That is in the experiment that got us into the whole thing. We really were not interested in the vW protein at the start. It was a good control, but we have not solved the problem that we set out to do, that is to identify the coagulant protein in these gels. I think we have got it going, but it is being done right now, this week. It has seemed like that for the past six months so I cannot really say that we are that much closer. It is a problem that is very important.

15

Factor VIIIC – immunology and activity

I. Peake

There are four essential aspects to the Factor VIII complex, which may be divided into two general areas. von Willebrand factor (vWf) is the term applied to the larger part of the complex, and biologically it may be assayed as ristocetin cofactor activity (VIIIR;Cof) which in some way reflects the in vivo activity in maintaining normal primary haemostasis (i.e. a normal bleeding time). Immunologically vWf is detected as Factor VIII related antigen (VIIIRAg). The relationship between VIIIR:Cof and VIIIRAg has been of particular importance in the recognition of the different types of von Willebrand's disease.

The second part of the Factor VIII complex is involved in the blood clotting system and is measured biologically as procoagulant or clotting Factor VIII (VIIIC) by clotting assays. The detection and measurement of antigens related to VIIIC (called VIIIC antigen or VIIICAg) has been developed over the last 2 years and the use of these assays, in conjunction with VIIIC assays is already producing some interesting data, particularly in relation to haemophilia.

ASSAY OF VIIICAg

VIIICAg may be measured by inhibitor neutralisation assay, but the techniques involved are technically difficult and the methods lack sensitivity. Immunoradiometric assays, both solid and fluid phase have been developed in several laboratories[1-3] and utilise antibodies to VIIIC obtained from human sources either from polytransfused haemophiliacs or from otherwise normal individuals with spontaneous inhibitors. All reports have shown good agreement between levels of VIIIC and VIIICAg in normal plasma. Unlike VIIIC, VIIICAg has also been shown to be present in normal serum at levels of approximately 70% of the corresponding plasma level. Of particular relevance is the stability of VIIICAg and its level in plasma has been shown to remain unaltered over 24 hours at 37°C, while that of VIIIC falls to 30% of the original value[4]. These results clearly suggest differences between the biological activity site and the antigenic sites detected by the anti VIIIC antibodies.

VIIIC AND VIIICAg IN HAEMOPHILIA

In the large majority of severe haemophiliacs both VIIIC and VIIICAg levels are undetectable. However, there are cases reported with low but detectable levels of VIIICAg in the order of 5 U/dl. The situation in mild haemophilia is more complex. Cases with up to 30 U/dl VIIIC and no detectable VIIICAg can be seen together with those with low VIIIC levels and normal VIIICAg (CRM + haemophilia). Others have comparable levels of the two activities, and thus types of haemophilia may soon be defined. Of particular interest is the possible variation of VIIICAg results obtained with different inhibitors. In practice, although inhibitors can give higher or lower VIIICAg levels, the differences are small, and the agreement between different assays surprisingly good. Certainly the diagnostic capability of different assays for VIIICAg appears to be equally good. However the results in mild haemophilia again confirm the view that the antigenic and biologically active sites, although related, are not identical.

VIIIC AND VIIICAg IN DIAGNOSIS AND RESEARCH

Carrier Detection In Haemophilia

Since the studies of Zimmerman et al.[5] the ratio of VIIIC to VIIIRAg has been used extensively for the detection of haemophilia carriers. Between 75% and 90% of obligate carriers have been shown to have a C/RAg ratio below the normal range. Preliminary data (Peake et al., unpublished observations) has shown that the ratio of VIIICAg to VIIIRAg may have more discriminatory power, largely because of the greater stability of VIIICAg when compared to VIIIC. These results, however, require confirmation.

The Detection Of Inhibitors Of VIIIC

Using the VIIICAg solid phase immunoradiometric assay it is possible to assay the inhibitor level in an unknown plasma. This is achieved by studying the effect on the binding of labelled antibody to antigen of prior incubation with the test material. Any antibodies present will reduce this binding and thus, by using a standard inhibitor plasma of known antibody titre (measured by clotting inhibitor assay using the Bethesda method), the titre of the unknown sample can be assessed. Preliminary results suggest results of the same order as the clotting assay, but with a sensitivity of 0.1 U/ml or less.

The Biochemical Relationship Between VIIIC, VIIICAg And VIIIRAg

This is an area where the VIIICAg assay will be of considerable importance since earlier studies of the relationship between VIIIC and VIIICAg have often suffered from the instability of VIIIC. Gel filtration studies have already suggested that in normal plasma some VIIICAg exists without associated VIIIC or VIIIRAg (Peake[6]). Similarly $Al(OH)_3$ has been shown to preferentially absorb VIIICAg from normal plasma, particularly if the plasma is lyophilised (Barrowcliffe et al., unpublished observations).

The Tissue Localisation And Synthesis Of VIIIC (VIIICAg)

VIIIRAg has been shown to be localised and synthesised by endothelial cells[7,8] and also to be present in platelets and synthesised by megakaryocytes[9]. However close examination of endothelial cells and platelets for the presence of VIIIC and VIIICAg have been entirely negative, as have studies on other tissues. The question of where VIIIC and VIIICAg are synthesised is still one of the major unresolved problems in the field of haemophilia.

REFERENCES

1.   Peake, I.R. and Bloom, A.L. (1978). Immunoradiometric assay of procoagulant factor VIII antigen in plasma and serum and its reduction in haemophilia. Lancet, 1, 473

2.   Lazarchick, J. and Hoyer, L.W. (1978). Immunoradiometric measurement of the factor VIII procoagulant antigen. J. Clin. Invest., 62, 1048

3.   Reisner, H.M., Barrow, E.S. and Graham, J.B. (1979). Radioimmuno-assay for coagulant factor VIII related antigen. Thrombosis Res., 14, 235

4.   Peake, I.R., Bloom, A.L. Giddings, J.C. and Ludlan, C.A. (1979). An immunoradiometric assay for procoagulant factor VIII antigen: results in haemophilia, von Willebrand's disease and fetal plasma and serum. Br. J. Haematol., 42, 269

5. Zimmerman, T.S., Ratnoff, O.D. and Littell, A.S. (1971). Detection of carriers of classic haemophilia using an immunologic assay for antihaemophilic factor. J. Clin. Invest., 50, 255

6. Peake, I.R. (1979). Factor VIII clotting antigens studied by immunoradiometric assay. Thrombosis Haemostasis, 42, 343

7. Bloom, A.L., Giddings, J.C. and Wilks, C.J. (1973). Factor VIII on the vascular intima: possible importance in haemostasis and thrombosis. Nature, New Biology, 241, 217

8. Jaffe, E.A., Hoyer, L.W. and Nachman, R.L. (1973). Synthesis of antihaemophilic factor antigen by cultured human endothelial cells. J. Clin. Invest., 52, 2757

9. Nachman, R., Levine, R. and Jaffe, E.A. (1977). Synthesis of factor VIII antigen by cultured guinea pig megakaryocytes. J. Clin. Invest., 60, 914

Discussion

Prof. Graham: Did you look at VIIIC and CAg^S, not as ratios of RAg but as independent entities in your carrier prediction?

The reason I ask the question is this. If someone does triplicate estimations and looks at the median, what you do is to throw out the outliers, so that looking at it that way one might be getting a very good estimate of VIIIC having thrown away the two bad values. I was astonished that there was not more differences than what you showed with the ratio, but in our experience the Factor VIII related antigen under the conditions that we examined our data did not seem to add very much information.

Dr. Peake: I took the data to a statistician with the idea of perhaps looking at the ratios. He did have a cursory look at the VIIIC and the VIIICAg on their own, but in his own words 'threw them out'. Presumably I can go back to him and ask him to do it again, but his initial analysis was done on the basis of ratios.

He did show quite clearly that seeing the patients 3 times considerably improved the discriminant compared with seeing them once, particularly from the point of view of VIIIC, as was to be expected from the variation problem.

Dr. Tuddenham: We do not see this phenomenon in patients with measurable clotting activity but no detectable VIIIC antigen.

Dr. Peake: I know, and we have discussed this. It is a possibility that these people who have 27 per cent VIIIC and no VIIICAg had only one antigenic site on the VIIICAg molecule which we were not detecting. But we checked for that by using it in the competing system by mixing test plasma with the label. In that situation, one site should bind the label and prevent it binding to the immobilised antigen. And in no cases have we ever found a level of less than 0.1 per cent CAg which had in effect a binding antibody. I have no evidence to show that any of ours were one-site antigens.

Dr. Tuddenham: The obligate carriers that were tested, are they the families who are C-antigen negative in your series?

Dr. Peake: The obligate carriers in that group are from the whole area of severe and mild haemophilia. We have not done the analysis of putting them into milds and severes.

Dr. Tuddenham: And at the C-antigen level ...... ?

Dr. Peake   That would be the split we would probably do, using the C-antigen level.

Dr. Ludlam: I was interested in Dr. Peake's data on absorption of CAg to aluminium hydroxide. Have you looked at the absorption of CAg in serum to aluminium hydroxide?

Dr. Peake: No, we have not.

Dr. Kernoff: Could you give your views on the nature of the Factor VIII related property which, when it is put into the patients with von Willebrands disease causes a rise in their level of VIIIC, where does that fit into the scheme of VIII-associated things?

Dr. Peake: If we look at severe von Willebrands disease, with no measurable VIII-related antigen, and a little bit, perhaps of VIIIC, we always get at VIIICAg result round about 5 or 6 per cent. So severe vW disease, homozygous vW disease, appear to have the ability to produce a small amount of VIIICAg. The argument would go, that when VIII-related antigen is infused, in some way it stimulates production of VIIIC or VIIICAg and that stimulated production continues on longer than the presence of VIII related antigen infused. That is the way I would look at it. The presence of a small amount of VIII-coag in severe vW disease would at least suggest that there is the ability to synthesise. Maybe it has a very short half-life, it is not stabilised, because there is no VIIIRAg there.

Prof. Stewart: I am a little disturbed by your figures. First, the one that interests us most is the one which overlaps the normal. It was not clear from your figure whether it was the same patient in your assay which was overlapping. Secondly, when you came to do the statistics, you seemed to have lost some of your patients. You started with 23 and the statistics were on 18.

Dr. Peake: The ones that overlap with C over RAg also overlap with CAg over RAg. I did not loose them, but my statistician, who is much stricter than I am, lost them because he felt that in one or two cases we had not been able to get 3 VIIIC assays at one time, and being a statistician, and not knowing the problems, he just thew them out. So that reduced it to 18. Then he did add that it did not matter whether 18 or 23. The results were equally as valid. I have a whole box full of slides which explains what he did, but I have given up on those because I do not understand them.

Prof. Stewart: So we do not give any extra help by doing this when we are stuck at the present time?

Dr. Peake: It is very discriminanting. Let me put it another way. If we take the ratio of 0.5 and 1, that is normal and carrier, if we look at the difference in likelihood ratio, that is that curve, for VIIIC over RAg, then the difference at 0.5 is about 200 times that at 1.0. The discrimination with the CAg over RAg is about 2,000 times. In other words, a value of 0.5 in a carrier using a CAg over RAg is a lot better discriminant from the normal than is a ratio of C over RAg. That is shown by the difference in steepness of those curves.

Prof. Stewart: It is all very well to say that the chances are 100:1 that someone is but my assay makes him 1,000:1. There really is no difference. It is in fact those people whom I cannot do - and you cannot help. Is that what you are trying to say?

Dr. Peake: I think it is marginally better in that, although the data does not show it, what Dr. Graham will add is that we take that figure, and then we combine it with the prior probability from the family tree to produce a final figure.

Dr. Chalmers: Do I understand from the little interplay between you and Dr. Graham that you do your assay 3 times, and then you take the median value of the 3 estimates and use that median value, so that you may very well finish up with a value for one estimate done one day and another estimate done another day, but they are the median values. Is that correct?

Dr. Peake: 'Yes, that is right.

Additional discussion of
Chapters 14 and 15

Dr. Rizza: Could I ask Dr. Hoyer about thrombin activation of
Factor VIII. This activiation is only detected in the one-stage FVIII assay?

Prof. Hoyer: We have only been following it in the one-stage assay.
That is right.

Dr. Rizza: It is said that the activiated Factor VIII can be
adsorbed by alumina. Do you have any ideas as to the mechanism of this
adsorption of the increased activity?

Prof. Hoyer: One would postulate, perhaps, that in the process of
fragmentation, that is associated with activation, that we are now changing
the physical properties of this coagulant protein and making it more
adsorbable. We see this in trying to do gel filtration studies in that we
cannot do a gel filtration on G-200 in the presence of standard buffers.
It gets lost. It gets adsorbed into the Sephadex - both the coagulant
activity and the coagulant protein measured immunologically if it has been
thrombin activitated, and we can only obviate that by doing the separations
in one-molar sodium chloride.

My feeling is that when the coagulant protein is activated, it gets
changed in a way that makes it stickier, makes it more susceptible to
electrostatic interactions, and that is probably why it now sits on
phospholipid and does its job.

Dr. Prentice: Would Dr. Hoyer speculate on VIIIC in vW disease.
Would he go along with the view that one has accelerated degradation of the

material due to the lack of a stabilising effect? What would his speculations be on this relationship?

Prof. Hoyer: They have to be very clearly labelled speculations because the experiments will be very hard to do. We get exactly the same results with the coagulant antigen assay. We always find maybe 2 or 3 per cent in the severe von Willebrand's patient, so that they have the genetic capacity as we know, and therefore they are probably making it. I do not think one can choose today among three alternatives. Either Factor VIII - related protein is stimulating synthesis, it is allowing escape from the cell in which it is synthesised into the plasma, or it is protecting it. Some studies that Dr. Weiss and I did years ago showed a definite protection of the small low-molecular weight Factor VIIIC by haemophilic plasma or Factor VIII related protein, so that I am attracted to that notion, but the mathematics are very hard, because the coagulant protein in the transfused vW patient stays up after the bulk of the Factor VIII related protein has gone. So either we are dealing with a super stabiliser, or that cannot be the whole story and it is more likely related to stimulation or escape from the cell.

To go back to Dr. Kernoff's point, the principle in the Factor VIII complex responsible for that rise can only be identified in a patient and therefore we are really left with the historical data. All of those materials that appear to stimulate the late response all now are known to contain Factor VIII related protein in a relatively native sense - haemophilic plasma, serum, as well as normal plasma, cryoprecipitate and so forth. So I think as we go back to that old data it supports the notion that it is the Factor VIII-related protein.

We also have the data from Bowie and Owen that in the perfused von Willebrand livers, the Factor VIII related protein seems to allow Factor VIII coagulant escape into the effluent, so it looks like that is the material but it will be very hard to prove in vivo.

Anonymous: Presumably the higher molecular weight polymers are primarily responsible for this apparent stimulant activity.

Prof. Hoyer: One would expect so, but we shall have to see.

Dr. Chediak: What effect does plasmin have on the complex.

Prof. Hoyer: We have not studied it directly. I can only comment on others' data that the coagulant protein is rather rapidly inactivated by plasmin. It is very sensitive, without an activation phase, while the Factor VIII related protein is relatively more resistant although it is degraded with loss of the larger polymers. I really do not have any primary data.

Prof. Stewart: It seems that the light fraction is the one we should be giving our Factor VIII deficient patients in the clinics, and yet it is the heavy fraction which we are getting down in the cryoprecipitate. We know it is effective, but the data we have been shown would suggest we should not do that, we should find the light fraction, the supernatant one.

Prof. Hoyer: If one could prepare material – as was discussed earlier in the proceedings – that has just the coagulant protein with small amounts on von Willebrand factor, and this isolated coagulant protein was more stable, yes, then I would agree that would be probably the best product. The problem is with present fractionation methods the most efficient way to get the coagulant protein is to take advantage of the fact that it sticks to the carrier, and both the alcohol separation methods and the cryoprecipitation methods take down the large fraction, so it is perhaps a historical accident that we get the large polymers even though they are not necessarily the best ones for coagulant activity. It is efficient, however.

16 Genetics of Factor VIII

J. Graham

My remarks about the genetics of Factor VIII consist of a few facts and a great deal of speculation. They go far beyond what is firmly established. My purpose is to erect a heuristic framework to accommodate the discoveries which I anticipate during the next few years. I am so uneasy about performing in this fashion for a group accustomed to conclusions based on extensive documentation that I should explain my epistemology.

Figure 1 summarises pictorially certain ideas about the nature of scientific research associated with a famous philosopher of science, Sir Karl Popper, and were discussed at length by him many years ago[1].

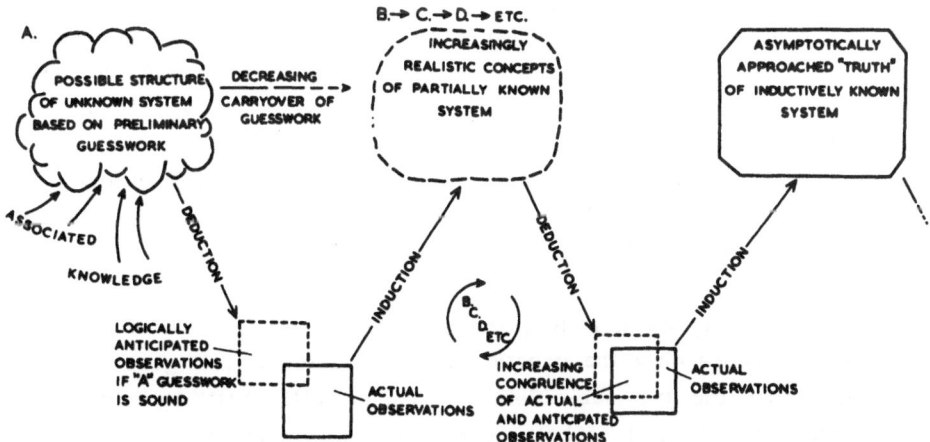

Figure 1   Cycles of deduction and induction leading from an initial idea to a firm hypothesis

[Research supported (in part) by a research grant (HL-06350) from the NIH]

The figure is an idealised description of the experimental process we use, but it illustrates how one's broodings lead to laboratory experiments which in turn modify one's ideas and lead to further experiments. These cycles of deduction and induction are repeated over and over, the initial hypothesis becoming highly refined in the process. As shown in the cloud at the upper left, the process begins with vague ideas drawn from a variety of sources which stimulate the investigator to create a working hypothesis. He then deduces that, if his hypothesis is correct, a certain experiment can be used to test it and does so, as shown in the lower left. The test may be decisively negative, causing the hypothesis to be rejected, or the observations may fit the hypothesis partially, suggesting that the scientist may be on the right track. Results which fit in part, provide new clues, and the scientist inductively modifies the hypothesis, as shown in the middle cloud in the upper part of the figure. The modified hypothesis then leads to a second series of experiments, which again, if they do not reject the hypothesis, refine the hypothesis further. This cyclic process is repeated until the original hypothesis is either discarded or refined to the point of establishment, perhaps as a "principle" or even a "law". My comments today will deal with matters which lie largely in the cloud at the top left of Figure 1 and the initial experiments which they suggest. This is because we are, in my judgment, at the very beginning of any real understanding of the genetics of Factor VIII. Progress lies, I believe, in adopting not only the techniques, but especially the method of molecular biology. Specifically, our problems require wide-open discussion and speculation to uncover the crucial experiments, followed by co-operative efforts to carry them out, because these experiments will be very difficult to carry out successfully. Those interested in the dynamics of the successes of molecular biology are urged to read Judson's fascinating history of the subject[2].

Now let me quickly provide you with the skeleton of my working hypothesis concerning the genetic contol of Factor VIII (Figure 2). I shall propose that the two sub-moieties of Factor VIII, VIIIRAg and VIIICAg, are under the control of both regulatory and structural genes, and that, because there are five distinguishable mutant phenotypes, at leat five genes are involved. The phenotypes to which I refer are listed at the bottom of the figure.

Before I go further, perhaps I should define the gene in terms suitable for my discussion.

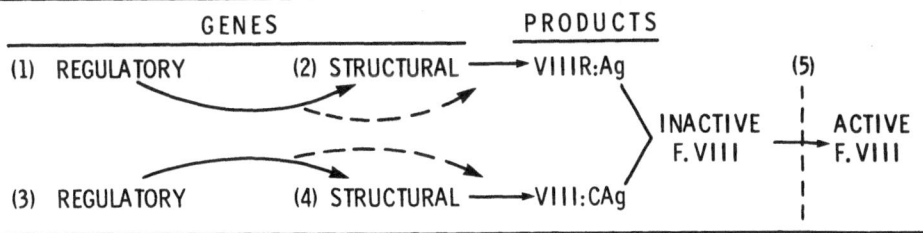

GENETIC CONTROL OF FACTOR VIII

Mutation Results in:

(1) Classical vWD
(2) "Atypical" vWD
(3) Dominant hemophilia A
(4) Recessive (X-linked) hemophilia A
(5) Combined deficiencies of Fs. V & VIII

Figure 2   The working hypothesis which is to be elaborated

Although it is an oversimplification, I shall define the gene as a linear, but not necessarily continuous, stretch of DNA. I shall regard genes as either structural or regulatory, although strictly speaking all genes are structural.

A structural gene shall be considered to be a stretch of DNA whose sequence contains the code for a peptide essential in normal physiology, e.g. globin, G-6-P-D or a blood clotting factor. A regulatory gene, on the other hand, shall be considered to be a stretch of DNA which contains the code for a product - nucleotide or a peptide - which functions to modify the rate of production, release, activation, transport or degradation of the product of a structural gene.

When dealing with a peptide of interest, there are several corollaries of these definitions that we should keep in mind. Until it is shown to be untrue, we should assume that a demonstrable change in the structure of a peptide indicates that there has been mutation of its structural gene. Mutation of a gene responsible for a post-translational modification will be regarded under our definition as a regulatory mutation, but structural change due to this mechanism is not always easily distinguished from a change in the primary sequence. The phenotypes resulting from mutation of structural genes may range from no alteration in physiology (silent mutation) to completely devastating syndromes, e.g. Lesch-Nyhan Syndrome, etc.

As shown in Figure 3, certain types of mutations of structural genes (frame shifts, deletions) may result in complete absence of a peptide (CRM$^-$ mutation). Mutations of this type cannot be distinguished phenotypically from mutations of regulatory genes with major effects, however, since no product may be detectable in either case. The demonstration that cross-reactive material is present (CRM$^+$) in a mutant phenotype showing reduced functional activity is, however, very informative. It shows that the reduction has resulted from mutation of a structural gene. Furthermore, if a mutation resulting in complete absence of a product maps at the same genomic position as a CRM$^+$ mutant, we may conclude that it is a CRM$^-$ mutation of the same structural gene.

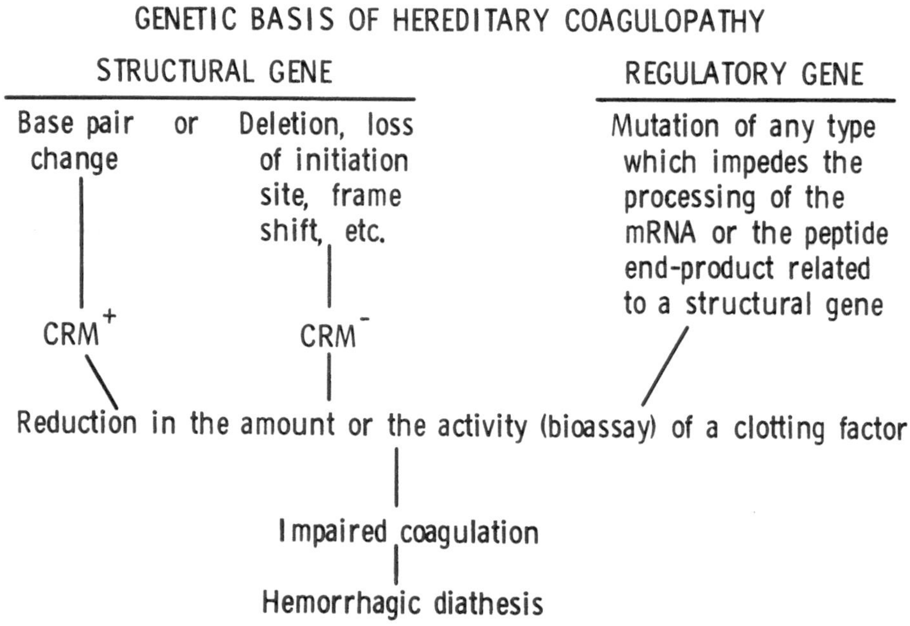

GENETIC BASIS OF HEREDITARY COAGULOPATHY

STRUCTURAL GENE	REGULATORY GENE

Base pair   or   Deletion, loss
change   of initiation
               site, frame
               shift, etc.

Mutation of any type which impedes the processing of the mRNA or the peptide end-product related to a structural gene

CRM$^+$ CRM$^-$

Reduction in the amount or the activity (bioassay) of a clotting factor

Impaired coagulation

Hemorrhagic diathesis

Figure 3   The genetic basis of an hereditary coagulopathy is assumed for our purposes to be mutation of a single gene, structural or regulatory

Mutation of a regulatory gene concerned with the production, release, transport, activation or degradation of the product of a structural gene, may cause either an increase or a decrease in the amount of end product. In the blood coagulation field the usual circumstances of ascertainment, i.e. observation of a bleeding tendency, imply that there has been a decrease in the amount of an end product. In several kindred with precocious thrombosis, however, an increase in Factor VIII activity has been reported[3], possibly representing an opposite type of regulatory change. Mutation of a regulatory gene usually implies no change in the structure of the end product, unless the gene in question is involved in a post-translational modification, such as addition of GLA residues[4]. The phenotypic hallmarks of a regulatory gene, except as noted above, are close parallelism between the amounts of biological and immunological activity of the end product and absence of qualitative differences between "wild type" and mutant end products. Another useful distinction is that most, but not all, structural genes are recessive while many regulatory genes are dominant.

Table 1   Events during peptide synthesis under genetic control

Location	Event
On the chromosome	Inactivation during development
At transcription	Multiplicity of chromosomal genes (gene reiteration) Extrachromosomal replication of genes (gene amplification)
Post transcription	Processing of mRNA Transport of mRNA Degradation of mRNA Attachment of mRNA Translation of mRNA
Post translation	Modification of peptides Storage of peptides Secretion of peptides Degradation of peptides

Should we expect to encounter regulatory genes related to the synthesis of clotting factor–Factor VIII? Table 1 contains a partial list of well-known events during peptide synthesis in eucaryotic cells during which the products or regulatory genes affect the amounts of end product coded by structural genes. Twelve such events are listed and there are many others; we may confidently assume that each event is controlled by well-defined regulatory genes. Since each event is under genetic control, it is probably the functional efficiencies of the "normal" variants of the various regulatory genes which we recognise in the phenotype as the quantitative effects of "modifier" genes. Thus many regulatory genes are involved in governing the expression of each structural gene, some having greater effects than others on the amount of the resulting peptide. If each regulatory gene for each step in protein synthesis were unique for each peptide, there would be twenty to a hundred times as many regulatory genes as structural genes. However, many of the regulatory genes probably serve a large number of structrual genes, the best example being the structural gene coding the DNA polymerase which transcribes all structural genes. Let me summarise by saying, yes, we should expect to encounter inherited deficiency phenotypes for Factor VIII resulting from mutation of regulatory genes.

I shall be using certain terms to refer to Factor VIII which grow out of the laboratory methods we use. Coagulant activity, the output of conventional Factor VIII bioassays, will be referred to as VIIIC. The antigenic activity related to coagulant Factor VIII will be referred to as VIIICAg (or CAg). Setting aside such esoteric matters as avidity and affinity of antibodies, I regard immunological assays for VIIICAg as reflecting rather closely the number of molecules of the product coded by the structural gene on the X chromosome; for this reason I shall also refer to "molecules of CAg". VIIIRAg (RAg) is the term I shall use to refer to an antigenic moiety related to Factor VIII which is coded on a chromosome other than the X chromosome. I assume that immunological assays for RAg give rather direct information about the number of molecules of RAg present. VIIIRWF, meaning Factor VIII related Willebrand factor (or ristocetin cofactor), is a bioassay closely related to RAg and expresses how well the RAg assists in the aggregation of platelets under certain conditions.

I find that it is necessary to have a definite concept about the nature of Factor VIII if I am to consider its genetics. My concept is shown in Figure 4, and I think this diagram represents the mainstream of thought among the biochemists who have studied Factor VIII. I conceive of RAg and CAg as separate and distinct peptides, which means that they must be coded by separate and distinct structural genes. This fits with our knowledge that the RAg locus is autosomal while the CAg locus is X-linked.

Thus we begin with at least two structural genes which are widely separated in the genome. The products of these loci associate in some fashion because the CAg and RAg activities are isolated together when plasma is fractionated. However, the antigenic moieties are separable in vitro at high salt concentrations[5,6] or by differential absorption with polyelectrolytes[7] or by filtration through certain Amicon membranes[8].

FACTOR VIII

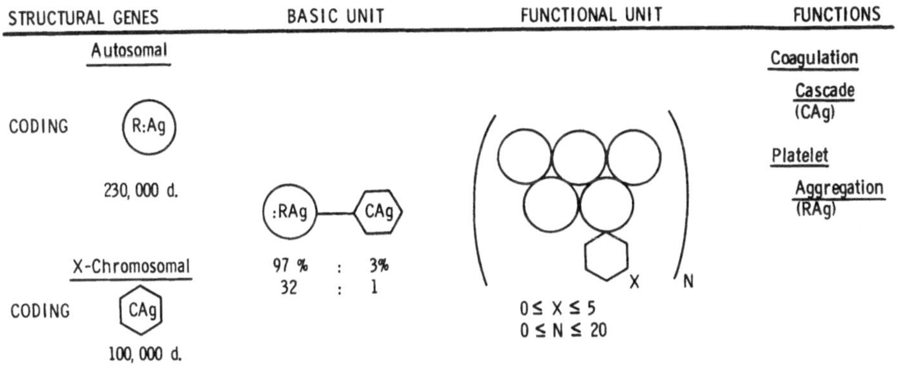

STRUCTURAL GENES	BASIC UNIT	FUNCTIONAL UNIT	FUNCTIONS

Autosomal

CODING (R:Ag)

230,000 d.

X-Chromosomal

CODING CAg

100,000 d.

:RAg — CAg

97 % : 3%
32 : 1

$0 \leq X \leq 5$
$0 \leq N \leq 20$

Coagulation
Cascade (CAg)

Platelet
Aggregation (RAg)

Figure 4 Working concept of the nature of Factor VIII

There is probably an intermediate polymer of RAg and CAg, possibly consisting of five RAgs and one CAg, which polymerises to polymers of very large size. It is likely that CAg must be transported by RAg in order to efficiently carry out its coagulant function, and it appears that the larger polymers containing RAg are more efficient in platelet aggregation than the smaller ones. CAg appears to be entirely inessential for platelet aggregation since VIIIRWF assays and bleeding time are normal in CRM⁻ haemophilia A. But the main point of this figure is that there must be at least one structural gene for RAg and one structural gene for CAg.

Now how might Factor VIII synthesis be controlled? We may begin with the two structural genes, and imagine the existence of at least one regulatory gene separately related to each. As I indicated earlier, I shall not only propose the existence of at least one regulatory gene directly controlling the output of RAg and another of CAg, but also that the product of a fifth gene must be present if CAg is to be fully active coagulationally.

Table 2, modified from[9], contains the evidence that there are at least 5 distinguishable mutant phenotypes involving Factor VIII. I might point out that there are probably at least two subtypes related to two of these major types. I am referring to CRM⁺ and CRM⁻ variants of X-linked haemophilia and vWD Types 2 and 2B. I am proposing provisionally that the X-locus for haemophilia and the locus for Type 2 vWD are the genes which code CAg and RAg respectively, because certain features of the mutant phenotypes suggest that they result from the mutation of structural genes.

Table 2   Distinguishable phenotypic variants of the factor VIII complex

	Chromosomal type	Phenotypic effect	Factor VIII Activities						Type of mutant gene
			C[1]	CAg[2]	RAg[3]	RWF[4]	VC[5]	VAg[6]	
1. Normal	----	----	+	+	+	+	+	+	----
2. Classic haemo A	X	Rec.	-	CRM⁺ CRM⁻ +	+	+	+	+	Struct.
3. Dominant haemo A	Auto/X	Dom.	-	-	+	+	+	+	Reg.
4. Classic vWD	Auto.	Dom.	-	-	-	-	+	+	Reg.
5. Atypical vWD	Auto.	Dom.	+	+*	±	-	+	+	Struct.
6. V-VIII deficiency	Auto.	Rec.	-	+	+	+	-	+	Reg.

* Personal communication, H.L. Grainick
(+)=normal activity, amount, or structure
(-)=greatly reduced amount or activity
(±)=partially reduced activity and abnormal
    immunoelectrophoretic migration

[1] = Factor VIII coagulant activity
[2] = Factor VIII coagulant antigen
[3] = Factor VIII-related antigen
[4] = Ristocetin cofactor activity
[5] = Factor V coagulant activity
[6] = Factor V antigenic activity

Since the matrix of Figure 6 contains six rows and nine columns and carries a very large amount of information, I shall go through it systematically pointing out the characteristics of each of the mutant phenotypes and explaining why I think each results from mutation of either a structural or a regulatory gene.

In Table 2 a plus mark (+) means that test results indicated either normal activity or a normal amount of substance depending upon whether the test was a bioassay or an immunological procedure. Minus (-) means either that there was a greatly reduced amount of biological activity or of an antigen. Plus/minus (±) means either that there was partial reduction in biological activity or that an abnormal product was demonstrable, depending upon whether a bioassay or an immunological assay had been used. The cryptic column headings have the following meanings: (i) C represents the bioassay for coagulant VIII, (ii) CAg the immunological assay for the coagulant moiety, (iii) RAg the immunological activity related to the Willebrand factor, (iv) RWF the bioassay for Willebrand factor (ristocetin co-factor), (v) VC represents the bioassay for Factor V, and (vi) VAg the immunological assay for the Factor V. Normals are scored as plus (+) in all six tests, as shown in the top line.

The second line indicates that classic haemophilia results from mutation of a gene on the X chromosome, a fact long known from segregation patterns. The mutant gene is known to be recessive, because the heterozygous mothers of haemophiliacs are only very rarely affected clinically, and then as the result of "extreme Lyonization"[10,11]. We may conclude that the gene is a structural gene because both CRM^+ and CRM^- variants are observed, the CRM^+ or CRM^- state being essentially uniform in the affected members of a single family, while VIIIRAg, VIIIRWF, VC and VAg are normal.

A second mutation producing the haemophilia A phenotype (third line) has been described in a single kindred[12]. The trait was dominant, having occurred in three generations of women in one family; a grandmother, a mother and grand-daughter. Their plasma VIIIC levels were reduced, CAgs being reduced in proportion, both assays in the 3-5% range. All other tests were normal. We do not know whether the mutated gene is on the X chromosome or an autosome because of the limited amount of genetic information, but we believe the phenotype to result from mutation of a regulatory gene because of the dominance of the phenotype and because the VIIIC and VIIICAg were reduced proportionally.

The classic variety of von Willebrand's disease (fourth line) results from mutation of a gene on an autosomal chromosome. It is dominant, since both male and female heterozygotes are similarly affected, and both sexes transmit to both sexes. There is reduction of all <u>four</u> of the Factor VIII activities, without reduction of the Factor V activities. We regard this phenotype as due to mutation of a regulatory gene because it is dominant and the RAg and RWF moieties are reduced in proportion to each other. The major ambiguity concerns why VIIIC and VIIICAg are also reduced in von Willebrand's disease. If, as proposed in Figure 4, RAg is the carrier of CAg and is normally present in great excess, CAg may have a much shorter half life and, therefore, a lower equilibrium level when RAg is reduced, even though the amount of CAg being produced in the cells of synthesis may be entirely normal. If correct, this explanation implies that the entire RAg pathway should be regarded as a physiological mechanism for regulating the level of CAg, a matter to which I shall return later.

I refer to the second type to von Willebrand's disease (line 5) as "atypical von Willebrand's disease". Others refer to it as vWD type 2[13-15]. I am suggesting that this phenotype results from mutation of the structural gene coding RAg, because VIIIC and VIIICAg seem to be entirely normal, and the amount of RAg is normal in unidimensional immuno-electrophoresis. The bioassays related to RAg, i.e. the ristocetin co-factor assays and bleeding time are abnormal, and crossed immunoelectrophoresis suggests that VIIIRAg may be either abnormal in size or in electrical charge, i.e. structurally. A second variant has been reported and designated vWD Type 2B[16]. This is consistent with the idea that Type 2 vWD results from mutation of a structural gene, since a prediction of such an hypothesis is that multiple "variants" should exist. I reserve the possibility that the products of both these genes are involved in post-translational modification of VIIIRAg which would cause me to regard them as regulatory genes. If this were correct, then phenotypes representing mutation of the structural gene have not yet been encountered and there is an additional regulatory gene in the RAg pathway to account for. Such a situation would require an even more elaborate working hypothesis than the one that I shall be proposing.

The fifth variant known to affect the Factor VIII complex (line 6) results from mutation of a rare autosomal gene. The abnormal phenotype in homozygotes is characterised by greatly reduced coagulant activities of

Factors V and VIII in the presence of normal amounts of CAg, RAg, RWF and VAg. The evidence suggests that the Factor VIII (and V) molecules are present in normal amounts but that a type of activation common to both has not occurred. I suspect that the phenotype results from mutation of a structural gene coding a product needed to make a post-translational modification (activation) of these two clotting factors, but there are many other possibilities (vide Table 1).

Now, two things remain to be attended to. The first is to pull all the ideas I have expressed into a working hypothesis. Then, a proposal is needed for testing the hypothesis.

Before I outline the hypothesis let me prepare you with two additonal ideas. The more important is that I shall introduce a new paradigm for thinking about Factor VIII. I am using the term "new paradigm" in Thomas R. Kuhn's sense of a revolutionary change in our way of thinking. I shall be considering what may be going on in the cells which synthesise CAg and RAg rather than these factors as we observe them in plasma. It is more difficult to think about Factor VIII in this fashion but our knowledge that <u>cells</u> make Factor VIII, forces us to ask <u>how</u> they do so. It is also more difficult to think about Factor VIII in this manner than fibrinogen or prothrombin, because the cells of synthesis of Factor VIII are not yet known. Available evidence suggests that RAg is probably synthesised in endothelial cells[17,18] and CAg in hepatocytes[19,20] and, possibly, other cells. But I am forced to beg the question of a complete cellular explanation, except to assume that all peptides are synthesised <u>intracellularly</u> <u>somewhere</u>! If, as seems likely, CAg and RAg are synthesised In different cells, there is the additional question of how and where they are brought together.

The second, and less important, idea is that I shall be describing the genes responsible for synthesising Factor VIII using the genetic nomenclature for blood coagulation suggested by a working party of the International Committee on Thrombosis and Haemostasis in 1973[21]. As shown in Table 3, they recommended that the coagulation genes be designated first by reference to the roman numeral designation of the factor concerned, then assigned arabic numerals in their order of discovery. Because of the genetic complexity of Factor VIII, I shall modify this further by using arabic one (1) for all the genes related to CAg and an arabic two (2) for all the genes related to RAg. Thus in my formulation the loci which mutate to produce CAg deficiency will be designated VIII-1 and the genes which mutate to produce RAg deficiency will be VIII-2. The working party also suggested that structural genes be designated aa and regulatory genes rr, while the superscript plus (+) be used to indicate the "wild type" or "usual" allele and minus (-) an abnormal allele when there is not a detectable product. Examples at the bottom of the figure give the genetic designations for the normal or usual genes consistent with the working hypothesis I shall propose.

Table 3   Genetic nomenclature for blood coagulation

Factor	Locus	Allele
I		aa^+ usual (normal) struct.
.		aa^- CRM^-, no product
.	-1	rr^+ usual (normal) reg.
VIII		
.	-2	rr reduction phenotype
.		rs " structural (CRM^+)
XIII	-3	rc " control (reg.)

Examples:
VIII-1aa$^+$ = Normal structural gene at haemophilia locus
VIII-1rr$^+$ = Normal gene at dominant haemophilia locus
VIII-2rr$^+$ = Normal gene at classical vWD locus
VIII-2aa$^+$ = Normal gene at RAg structural locus

Figure 5 is arranged to show synthesis of Factor VIII. It takes into account that peptide synthesis is intracellular while the factors being studied are extra-cellular, i.e. in plasma. The figure also separates the CAg and RAg pathways. The figure is drawn to represent Factor VIII synthesis in a normal individual, although for simplicity the individual's genome is indicated as haploid rather than diploid!

The structural genes are designated aa^+ and the regulatory genes rr^+. The pathway for CAg synthesis is shown horizontally in the centre, the CAg locus ($1aa^+$) being the starting point. The dominant haemophilia locus, 1rr$^+$, is shown by broken arrows as controlling either the transcription, translation, transportation, secretion, etc. of CAg. The RAg pathway is shown vertically on the right, 2aa$^+$ being the structural or Type 2 vWD locus. The regulatory gene which mutates to produce classical vWD (2rr$^+$) is pictured by broken arrows as exerting its effect through transcription, translation or secretion, etc. RAg and CAg are brought together somewhere and CAg is activated by the product of the V–VIII locus either intracellularly or in plasma. By now, you have probably realised that a lifetime might be required to carry out the experiments suggested by this working hypothesis.

GENETIC CONTROL OF FACTOR VIII

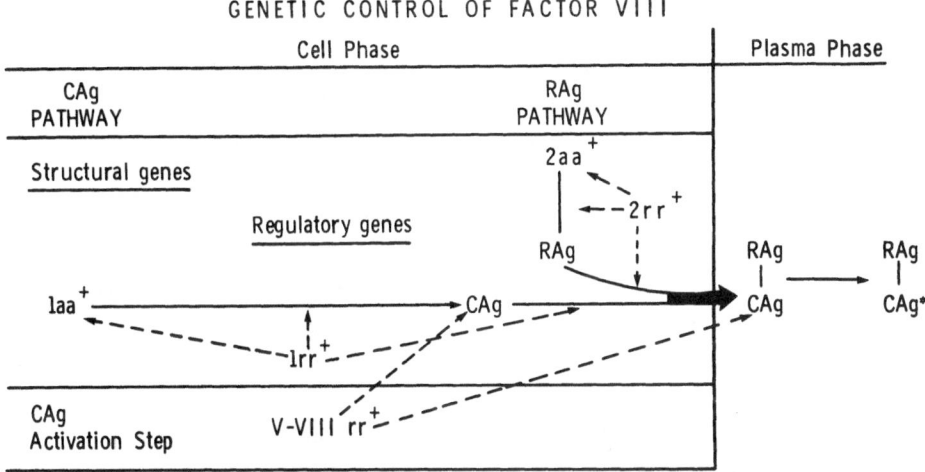

Figure 5   Elaborated working hypothesis concerning the genetic control of human blood coagulation Factor VIII.   The activities thought to take place intra-cellularly are contained within the heavy frame on the left.   The known physiological functions of Factor VIII occur in circulating blood and are indicated on the right outside the frame

We have now reached the point of considering what might constitute a critical test of the hypothesis.   Three possible approaches suggest themselves.   We might either discover and sequence the critical DNA, isolate and determine the sequence of the critical peptides, or proceed genetically.   Since I am geared to genetic studies, I shall leave the molecular biology to others, and suggest genetic tests of the hypothesis as it pertains to VIIIRAg.   The tests are complex and laborious and success is by no means assured, but the results might be decisive.   Both linkage studies of pedigrees transmitting vWD and somatic cell genetic studies of endothelial cells are required, and as I hinted earlier, they will probably require the co-operation of many laboratories and investigators. I doubt that geneticists who are struggling with this problem are going to be "scooped", except possibly by those who are attempting to clone the Factor VIII gene. Rumour has named three such groups in the USA alone, not surprising in view of the fantastic progress in molecular biology described in a recent issue of "Science"[22] and the rumoured $40 x 10^6 market for Factor VIII concentrate.

The genetic strategy is shown in Figure 6. All cells contain the genetic information to synthesise RAg but endothelial cells appear to produce it in great quantities. As shown on the right, it might be possible to assign the expression of RAg to a specific human chromosome using the techniques of somatic cell genetics. As shown on the left, pedigree studies of families with von Willebrand's disease might localise the vWD genes by linking the mutant genes to polymorphic markers whose chromosomal locations are known. It will be important to do pedigree studies on families with both classic and atypical vWD, since a difference between them would show that these genes are at separate locations. If successful, this strategy might tell us whether there is a single or whether there are multiple vWD loci.

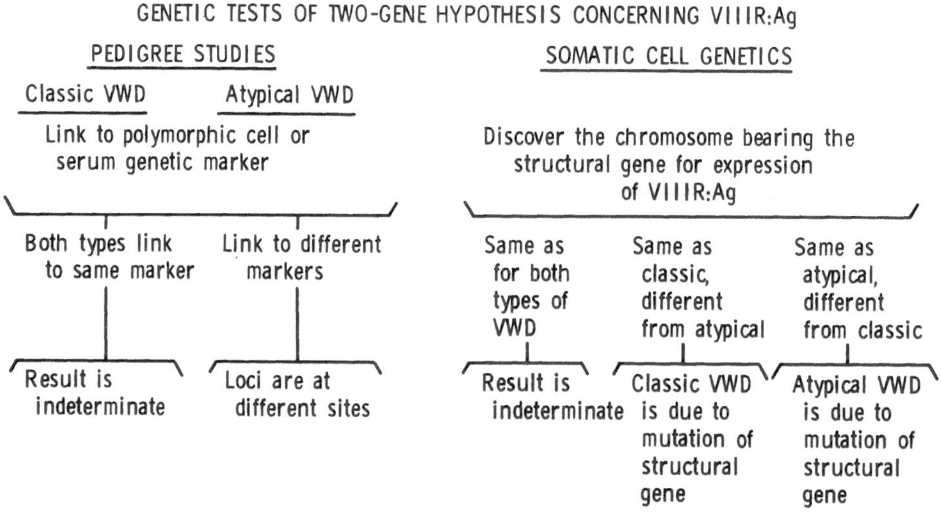

GENETIC TESTS OF TWO-GENE HYPOTHESIS CONCERNING VIIIR:Ag

PEDIGREE STUDIES		SOMATIC CELL GENETICS		
Classic VWD	Atypical VWD			
Link to polymorphic cell or serum genetic marker		Discover the chromosome bearing the structural gene for expression of VIIIR:Ag		
Both types link to same marker	Link to different markers	Same as for both types of VWD	Same as classic, different from atypical	Same as atypical, different from classic
Result is indeterminate	Loci are at different sites	Result is indeterminate	Classic VWD is due to mutation of structural gene	Atypical VWD is due to mutation of structural gene

Figure 6   The strategy of a genetic test of the hypothesis that synthesis of VIIIRAg is controlled by genes at more than a single locus

As it happens, my colleagues and I have been proceeding down both of these tracks for several years, with modest success. Dr. Emily Barrow is leading our attempt to link the vWD loci to polymorphic cell and serum markers by pedigree studies[23], while Dr. Cora-Jean Edgell is attempting to identify the human chromosome containing the gene responsible for expression of VIIIRAg, using hybrids between mouse cell lines and human endothelial cells[24]. Both types of research are very difficult. The pitfalls are many, and results emerge with tantalising slowness.

A poet produced some lines which seem to me to express my attitude towards the difficult types of research we are now becoming involved in. His verse, of course, meant something entirely different to him than it does to me, but I am pleased to find myself in any sort of harmony with such a great poet. I am sure that you will remember these lines from Alexander Pope's, "Essay on Man":

> "Awake, my St. John! Leave all meaner things
> To low ambition and the pride of Kings.
> Let us, since life can little more supply
> Than just to look about us and to die,
> Expatiate free o'er all this scene of man;
> A mighty maze! But not without a plan."

REFERENCES

1. Popper, K.R. (1959). The Logic of Scientific Discovery. (London: Hutchinson)

2. Judson, H.F. (1979). Eighth Day of Creation: Makers of the revolution in molecular biology. (New York: Simon-Schuster)

3. Penick, G.D., Dejanov, I.I., Reddick, R.L. and Roberts, H.R. (1966). Predisposition to intravascular coagulation. Thromb. Diath. Haemorrh., Suppl. 21, 543

4. Chung, K.S., Bezaud, A., Goldsmith, J.C., McMillan, C.W., Menache, D and Roberts, H.R. (1979). Congenital deficiency of blood clotting factors II, VII, IX, and X. Blood, 53, 776

5. Weiss, H.J., Phillips, L.L. and Rosner, W. (1972). Separation of sub units of antihaemophilic factor (AHF) by agarose gel chromatography. Thromb. Diath. Haemorrh., 28 212

6. Owen, W.G. and Wagner, R.H. (1972). Antihaemophilic factor: Separation of an active fragment following dissociation by salts or detergents. Thromb. Diath. Haemorrh., 28, 502

7. Johnson, A.J., MacDonald, V.E., Semar, M. et. al.(1978). Preparation of the major plasma fractions by solid-phase polyelectrolytes. J. Lab. Clin. Med., 92, 194

8. Newman, J., Harris, R.B. and Johnson, A.J. (1976). Molecular weights of antihaemophilic factor and von Willebrand factor proteins in human plasma. Nature, 263, 612

9. Graham, J.B. (1980). Genetic control of factor VIII. Lancet, 1, 340

10. Graham, J.B., Barrow, E.S. and Elston, R.C. (1975). Lyonisation in haemophilia: a cause of error in direct detection of heterozygous carriers. Ann. N.Y. Acad. Sci., 240, 141

11. Graham, J.B. Miller, C.H., Reisner, H.M., Elston, R.C. and Olive, J.A. (1976). The phenotypic range of haemophilia A carriers. Am. J. Human Genet., 28, 482

12. Graham, J.B., Barrow, E.S., Roberts, H.R., et. al. (1975). Dominant inheritance of haemophilia A in three generations of women. Blood, 46, 175

13. Peake, I.R., Bloom, A.L. and Giddings, J.C. (1974). Inherited variants of factor VIII related protein in von Willebrand's disease. N. Engl. J. Med., 291, 113

14. Gralnick, H.R., Coller, B.S. and Sultan, Y. (1974). Studies of human factor VIII/von Willebrand factor protein III: Qualitative defects in von Willebrand's disease. J. Clin. Invest., 56, 814

15. Ardaillou, N., Girma, J.P., Meyer, D., et. al. (1978). "Variants" of von Willebrand's disease. Demonstration of a decrease in antigenic reactivity by immunoradiometric assay. Thromb. Res., 12, 817

16. Ruggeri, Z.M. Pareti, F.I., Mannucci, P.M. et. al. (1980). Heightened interaction between platelets and factor VIII/von Willebrand factor in a new subtype of von Willebrand's disease. N. Engl. J. Med., 302, 1047

17. Jaffe, E.A., Hoyer, L.W. and Nachman, R.L. (1974). Synthesis of von Willebrand factor by cultured human endothelial cells. Proc. Natl. Acad. Sci. (USA), 71, 1906

18. Shearn, S.A.M., Peake, I.R., Giddings, J.C., Humphrys, J. and Bloom, A.L. (1977). The characterisation and synthesis of antigens related to factor VIII in vascular endothelium. Thromb. Res., 11, 43

19. Marchioro, T.L., Hougie, C., Ragde, H. et. al. (1969). Organ homografts for haemophilia. Transplantation Proc., 1, 316

20. Owen, C.A., Bowie, E.J.W. and Fass, D.N. (1979). Generation of factor VIII coagulant activity by isolated, perfused, neonatal pig livers and adult rat livers. Brit. J. Haematol., 43, 307

21. Graham, J.B., Barrett, D.A., Blomback, B. et. al. (1973). A genetic nomenclature for human blood coagulation. Thromb. Diath. Haemorrh., 30, 1

22. "Recombinant DNA" (1980). Science, 209, 1319

23. Goldin, L.R., Elston, R.C., Miller, C.H. and Graham, J.B. (1981). Genetic analysis of von Willebrand's disease in two large pedigrees: a multivariate approach. Am. J. Med. Genet., (In press)

24. Edgell, C-J.S., Reisner, H.M. and Graham, J.B. (1981). Endothelial hybrids and suppression of factor VIII related antigen expression. Brit. J. Haematol., (In press)

Discussion

Prof. Bloom: I would basically agree with what you say. What I am not too sure about, and what I think nobody is really sure about is what you actually mean by classical von Willebrand's disease and atypical von Willebrand's disease. By classical vW disease if you mean people with prolonged bleeding time, and corresponding levels of the other measurements, then many of these patients will in fact be atypical.

Prof. Graham: What I mean precisely is that there must be mutation to the structural genes and there must be mutations to the regulatory mechanism. I am taking the working position that one of these is structural and the other is regulatory. If that is true, then there is a clear distinction between them. If it is not true, both of them may be regulatory and the structural gene may yet not have been discovered. It is possible that it may be a long time before we can make this distinction, but I would make my distinctions about vW disease at a very fundamental level, as fundamental as possible, as genetic as possible, and I would start by saying is it a regulatory phenomenon or is it a structural phenomenon? Beyond that you can go back and talk about sequence, what are the problems, what are the sequences and so on. In the case of the regulatory mutation one has got to discover a meaning, how does it function? Could it function anyway? Transcription? Transportation? Processing? It does not follow necessarily that they are not different regulatory mutations being seen in von Willebrand's disease operating at different places in the pattern.

Prof. Bloom: This has been put forward, so since the endothelium will also make plasminogen activator, it may be there is an abnormal proteolysis which would fit in with that view.

Dr. Colvin: If the hypothesis is true, and if dominant haemophilia breeds true, does that not mean it must be autosomal?

Prof. Graham: You would likely have a little stronger evidence than that; at least 3 generations who were exactly alike. Incidentally they have a very revealing problem. They have Factor VIIIC and CAg, and have very little problem.

Dr. Colvin: If it really is X-linked, then surely ....

Prof. Graham: You might think that it is. If we think about it, the whole RAg pathway is a regulatory system, regulating CAg production. Looked at on a physiological level, I just do not know. It is unfortunate that we cannot do the right experiments.

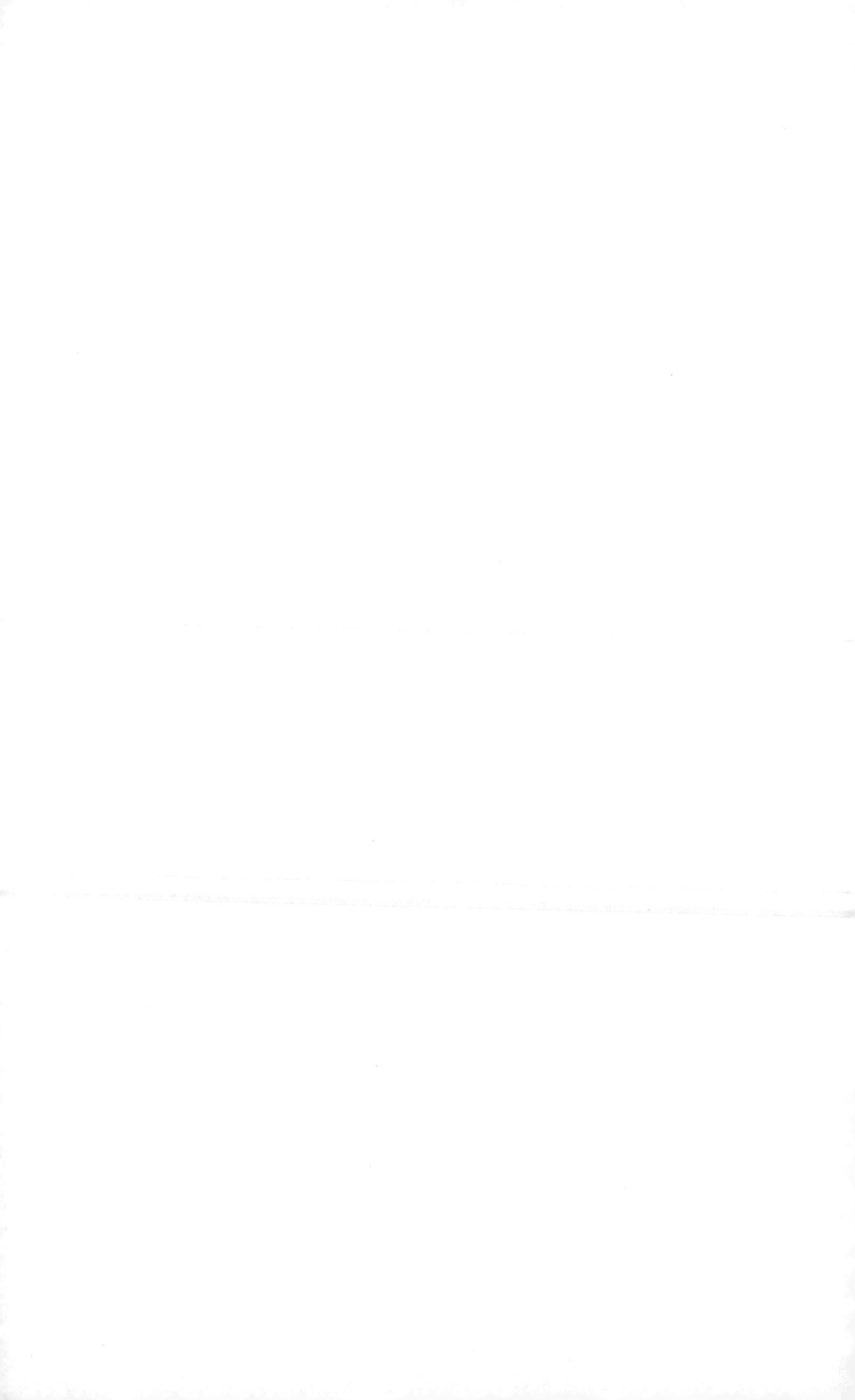

17 Prenatal diagnosis of haemophilia A and Christmas disease

R. Mibashan and C. Rodeck

Because of the X-linked recessive inheritance of both forms of haemophilia, the chance that a pregnant carrier's male foetus will be affected is 1 in 2, with a severity that is characteristic of that family's haemophilia.

Despite modern advances, haemophilia still makes heavy inroads on the physical, emotional and economic resources of those affected, their families and the whole community. Accordingly some carriers, whether proven or presumptive, are unwilling to bear a haemophilic son and take steps to avoid pregnancy or to terminate it if the foetus is male. At least 50% of these selectively aborted male foetuses are normal, and such mothers, in addition to undergoing the many-sided trauma of needless abortion, are unable to have normal boys.

Prenatal diagnosis aims at distinguishing between normal and haemophilic male foetuses, so that only the latter are aborted if the parents so wish. Two prerequisites, both recently attained, have made this objective possible: (1) a reliable method for obtaining pure foetal blood[1,2] and (2) the co-ordinated application of carefully standardised Factor VIII and IX assays to these small foetal samples[3-8].

PATIENTS AND METHODS

Preliminary

The clinical and laboratory details of the 'patient' and her affected relatives are critically reviewed, and care is taken to ensure that she receives full genetic counselling. While assessment of her probability of being a carrier by laboratory tests and pedigree analysis is a useful exercise[9,10], we have been impressed by the motivation of prospective mothers wishing to avoid bearing a haemophilic son when they have severely affected close relatives. Undue reliance should not be placed on carrier detection tests, with their inherent error of around 10%[11], in advising women at risk about prenatal diagnosis.

Amniocentesis is performed at 15 weeks under ultrasound guidance, to determine the foetal sex; great care must be taken to avoid red cell leakage into the amniotic fluid, as subsequent fetoscopy may be difficult or even impossible. If the foetus is male, the mother is admitted for fetoscopy at about 19 weeks.

Foetal Blood Sampling

The maternal Factor VIII or IX clotting activity is always assayed prior to fetoscopy to exclude a dangerously low level, relevant particularly if a termination of pregnancy ensues. However, replacement with cryoprecipitate or plasma was only deemed necessary once in 50 patients.

Fetoscopy is performed under sedation and local anaesthesia, using a Dyonics Needlescope. It's shaft is 15 cm long and the bore 1.7 mm, while the cannula through which it fits has an oval cross-section of 2.2 x 2.7 mm and an operating channel which admits a flexible 26- or 27-gauge blood-sampling needle. The site of introduction of trocar and cannula is selected with the greatest care during a real-time ultrasound scan performed under sterile conditions. The best site for foetal blood sampling is an umbilical vessel just above the placental insertion of the cord; here pure foetal blood can be aspirated from within the vessel lumen, haemostasis is good (even in haemophilic foetuses) and the chance of penetrating the intervillous space and causing foeto-maternal haemorrhage is low[2,7].

Immediately before puncture, the blood sampling needle is flushed with a sterile, isotonic citrate-saline solution to exclude amniotic fluid, which might initiate clotting during sampling or accelerate the assay times[5,12]. The vessel having been punctured under direct vision, serial amounts of 150-200 µl of pure foetal blood are withdrawn into a graduated 1ml plastic syringe, using a new syringe for each aliquot of blood. Into a tiny, calibrated polystyrene tube containing 100 µl of 36 mmol/l trisodium citrate-barbitone buffer, 100 µl of foetal blood is delivered, the rest of each aliquot going into EDTA and heparin. A combined cell counter and particle-size analyser (Coulter 'Channelyzer') shows within seconds that there is no maternal blood present (foetal red cells having a much larger MCV) and that successive blood samples have a constant haematocrit in the expected range, thus excluding even small amounts of variable dilution by amniotic fluid.

Four to six aliquots, i.e. up to 900 μl of foetal blood, are usually taken.

Coagulant Assays

After an hour's wait on ice, the samples are centrifuged and one-stage assays of Factors VIIIC and IXC are performed on the supernatant[5]. Factor VIIIRAg is also measured by the Laurell method. A correction is applied for the initial 1 in 2 dilution in citrate-buffer at fetoscopy.

Immunoradiometric assay of foetal Factor VIIIC antigen (VIIICAg). Blood samples from all foetuses at risk of haemophilia A were assayed for Factor VIIICAg by Peake and Bloom in Cardiff[5,13].

Diagnostic Patients And Controls

Pure foetal blood from 40 non-haemophilic foetuses undergoing fetoscopy for other reasons was used to determine control values. Fifty consecutive patients, two with a twin pregnancy, who sought prenatal diagnosis are reported here; 46 were at risk of haemophilia A and 4 of haemophilia B. The haemophilia A carriers were assigned to one of three groups of carrier probability according to the combined odds derived from their pedigree analysis and laboratory data[9,10,14]; 13 were obligate carriers (probability = 1); 28 were rated strongly putative (p = 0.5 - 0.99); and 5 were putative (p equal to or less than 0.25).

RESULTS

Table 1 shows the plasma clotting factor levels in a control group of foetal blood samples.

Of the 47 foetuses (in 46 patients) at risk of haemophilia A, 32 proved to be normal. A 33rd was found to have a massive encephalocele and a reduced VIIIC level, but compared with affected relatives it was not regarded as having haemophilia.

Table 1   Normal plasma levels of foetal factor VIII and IX[*]

	Gestation (weeks)	Haematocrit	VIIIC U/dl	VIIICAg[@] U/dl	VIIIRAg U/dl	IXC U/dl
Mean	19.2	0.37	45[r]	23	57[r]	8.5
SD	1.7	0.03	12	8	13	1.8
Range	16–23	0.33–0.43	25–89	11–43	41–103	5.9–12.8

[*] n = 40
[@] VIIICAg assays performed by Peake & Bloom (n = 20)
[r] Correlation r = 0.74; p < 0.001

The results in the 33 unaffected foetuses are shown in Table 2. This group includes twin males, from each of whom pure foetal blood was obtained through a single uterine insertion and trans-septal sampling of the second twin.

Table 2   Normal prenatal tests in 33 male foetuses at risk of haemophilia A[a,b,c]

	Gestation (weeks)	Hct[x]	Fetoscopy			Newborn[*,@]		
			VIIIC[x]	VIIICAg	VIIIRAg	VIIIC	VIIICAg	VIIIRAg
Mean	19.8	0.36	44	24	55	134	114	133
SD	1.6	0.03	10	9	10			
Range	16–24	.30–.42	31–81	11–46	34–73			

[a] including one pair of twins
[b] Assays in U/dl
[c] Carrier status: 8 obligate; 20 strongly putative; 5 putative
[*] Cord or neonatal sample
[@] Excludes: 3 still pregnant and 2 unrelated terminations
[x] Excludes one sample diluted 1 : 1.5 with amniotic fluid

The results in the 33 unaffected foetuses are shown in Table 2. This group includes twin males, from each of whom pure foetal blood was obtained through a single uterine insertion and trans-septal sampling of the second twin.

The measurement of foetal Factor VIII by both bioassay (VIIIC) and IRMA (VIIICAg) resulted in 100% overall diagnostic accuracy to date, which might not have occurred using one method alone: (a) Two normal foetuses belonged to a kindred whose affected members were CRM[+] with respect to VIIICAg; their normal coagulant assays dispelled the possibility

Table 3   Abnormal prenatal tests in 14 male foetuses at risk of haemophilia A[(a)]

Patient	Carrier status	Weeks	Hct	Fetoscopy VIIIC	Fetoscopy VIIICAg	Fetoscopy VIIIRAg	Abortus VIIIC	Abortus VIIICAg
H1	++	22	.43	3	0.1	57	1	0.1
H2	++	19	.36	2	0.1	52		0.1
H3	Obligate	20	.33	6[b]	0.1	55		3[b]
H4	Obligate	19	.36	1	9[c]	55		10[c]
H5	Obligate	20	.34	1	5[c]	70	1	
H6	++	20	.37	1	0.1	59	T	T
H7	++	19	.34	1	0.1	59		0.1
H8	Obligate	17	.35	1	0.1	35	T	T
H9	++	19	.34	1	0.1	50		0.1
H10	++	20	.35	1	0.1	46	1	0.1
H11	++	19	.36	1	0.1	41		0.1
H12	Obligate	19	.34	1	20[c]	39	1	22[c]
H13	++	18	.33	1	0.1	36	T	T
H14	++	19	.42	1	0.1	47	SIT	
	Mean	19.3	.36			50		
	SD	1.1	.03			10		

[a] Plasma assays in U/dl
[b] Mildly affected family
[c] CRM[+] family (H4 & 5 separate pregnancies in same carrier)
T Terminated abroad (no sample)
SIT Selective intrauterine termination of one twin

of false-normal IRMA values. (b) By contrast, one normal foetus in Table 2 yielded blood diluted 2.5-fold with aminotic fluid, owing to obscure vision caused by old blood from the amniocentesis. The VIIIC assay was thus unsafe, and a normal VIIICAg (in a CRM$^-$ kindred) established the foetal diagnosis.

Altogether 28 non-haemophilic babies have been born, including the twins, while 3 carriers are still pregnant at the time of writing; 2 of the 33 foetuses were aborted for reasons unconnected with haemophilia. Haemophilia A was diagnosed in 14 of the 47 foetuses at risk.

Pure foetal blood was obtained fetoscopically in every case, and there was good agreement between the 2 AHF assay methods, except in 3 foetuses who were CRM$^+$; in at least one of them (H12) and probably a second (H4), the immunoassay would not have enabled recognition of haemophilia, thus highlighting the importance of being able to measure coagulant Factor VIIIC. The findings were confirmed in the 10 available abortuses (and were congruent in the other 4).

Patient H14 had unlike twins; only the male was tested, found to be affected, and selectively terminated by a new technique[15]. The sister foetus is developing normally and awaits delivery.

Table 4   Relation between 46 foetal tests and carrier status (haemophilia A)

Carrier* status	Total number	Expected no. of carriers	Haemophilic foetuses expected	Haemophilic foetuses observed
Obligate	12	12	6	5
Putative ++ (0.5 or more)	29	14-29	7-14	9
Putative + (0.25 or less)	5	1	<1	0

* Excluding one foetal malformation (see text)

Table 4 reflects the predictive value of the prenatal assays, when these are analysed in terms of the assigned carrier status. It explains why the proportion of affected foetuses (14/46) is appreciably less than the 50% expected if all the carriers had been obligate, and illuminates the 'reprieve' rate among male foetuses of mothers who are unwilling to bear a haemophilic child.

Christmas Disease

Prenatal diagnosis of haemophilia B has lagged behind that of haemophilia A partly because it is less prevalent and also because the blood sampling and assay requirements are even more stringent in view of the normally low Factor IX levels.

Four foetuses were at risk of haemophilia B. One mother was an obligate carrier, the others strongly putative (pedigree probability 0.5 or 0.67 and reduced IXC levels in mid-pregnancy).

Table 5   Four male foetuses at risk of haemophilia B

Patient	Carrier status	Weeks	Fetoscopy*		Newborn
			Hct	IXC(U/dl)	IXC(U/dl)
B1	++	20	0.32	12.3	40
B2	Obligate	19	0.35	7.9	35
B3	++	22	0.34	9.4	45
B4	++	20	0.38	6.6	normal[+]

* Control foetal IXC   Mean   8.5 U/dl (S.D. 1.8)   (n = 40)

Range   5.9 - 12.8 U/dl

[+] Assayed abroad - value not stated

Plasma IXC levels were normal in all 4 foetuses and 4 healthy boys have since been delivered normally.

At the time of writing a 5th foetus was recognised prenatally to have haemophilia B, and this was confirmed after elective termination[16].

A sensitive IRMA for Factor IXAg has been reported by Holmberg et al.[8], capable of distinguishing normally low foetal levels from CRM$^-$

haemophilia B; this elegant assay is inapplicable to CRM^+ cases, however, whose incidence in Christmas disease is higher than in haemophilia A.

Table 6 shows the subsequent course of pregnancy in those studied. There were no maternal or foetal complications except 2 premature deliveries (i.e. earlier than 37 weeks), resulting in normally maturing babies. There were no incorrect diagnosis.

Table 6   Outcome of pregnancy after prenatal tests

Number of pregnancies	50
Number of foetuses	51
Pure foetal blood obtained in	50
termination (a) Haemophilia	14
(b) Other causes	2
Pregnancies continued	35

Normal deliveries	30
Not yet delivered	3
Pre-term labour	2
Maternal complications	0
Accidental abortions	0
Incorrect diagnosis	0

CONCLUSION

Prenatal diagnosis of the haemophilias has been shown to be a highly accurate investigation in clinical practice. Pure foetal blood can be obtained from virtually all foetuses, enabling Factor VIIIC and IXC bioassays to be performed and ensuring that no exclusions from diagnosis need occur because of CRM-positivity in immunoradiometric assay systems. The more complex IRMA techniques offer valuable confirmation in CRM^- cases, or an alternative diagnostic tool if the foetal samples should be spoiled by dilution or activiation. While fetoscopy carries a potential foetal risk, this can be kept encouragingly low, and the diagnostic error rate has been nil. Prenatal diagnosis is a valuable option for families who wish to utilise it.

REFERENCES

1. Rodeck, C.H. and Campbell, S. (1978). Sampling pure foetal blood by fetoscopy in second trimester of pregnancy. Br. Med. J., 2, 728

2. Rodeck, C.H. (1980). Fetoscopy guided by real-time ultrasound for pure fetal blood samples, fetal skin samples and examination of fetus in utero. Br. J. Obstet. Gynaecol., 87, 449

3. Firshein, S.I., Hoyer, L.W., Lazarchick, J., et. al. (1979). The prenatal diagnosis of classic haemophilia. N. Engl. J. Med., 300, 937

4. Mibashan, R.S., Rodeck, C.H., Thumpston, J.K., et. al. (1979). Prenatal plasma assay of fetal factors VIII and IX. Br. J. Haematol., 41, 611

5. Mibashan, R.S., Rodeck, C.H., Thumpston, J.K., et. al. (1979). Plasma assay of fetal factors VIIIC and IX for prenatal diagnosis of haemophilia. Lancet, 2, 1309

6. Peake, I.R., Bloom, A.L., Giddings, J.C. and Ludlam, C.A. (1979). An immunoradiometric assay for procoagulant factor VIII antigen. Results in haemophilia, von Willebrand's disease and fetal plasma and serum. Br. J. Haematol., 42, 269

7. Mibashan, R.S., Peake, I.R., Rodeck, C.H., et. al. (1980). Dual diagnosis of prenatal haemophilia A by measurement of fetal factor VIIIC and VIIIC antigen (VIIICAg). Lancet, 2, 994

8. Holmberg, L., Gustavii, B., Cordesius, E., et. al. (1980). Prenatal diagnosis of haemophilia B by an immunoradiometric assay of factor IX. Blood, 56, 397

9. Memorandum: Methods for the detection of haemophilia carriers. (1977). Bull. Wld. Hlth. Org., 55, 675

10. Graham, J.B. (1979). Genotype assignment (carrier detection) in the haemophilias. In: Rizza, C.R. (ed.). Clinics in Haematology - Congenital Coagulation Disorders, Vol 8, pp. 115-46. (London: W B Saunders Co. Ltd.)

212

11. Ratnoff, O.D., and Jones, P.K. (1977). The art of betting: Which of a bleeder's female relatives is a carrier? Ann. Intern. Med., _89_, 281

12. Yaffe, E., Eldor, A., Hornshtein, E. and Sadovsky, E. (1977). Thromboplastic activity of amniotic fluid during pregnancy. Obstet. Gynaecol., _50_, 454

13. Peake, I.R. and Bloom, A.L. (1978). Immunoradiometric assay of procoagulant factor VIII antigen in plasma and serum and its reduction in haemophilia. Lancet, _1_, 473

14. Mibashan, R.S., Thumpston, J.K., Rodeck, C.H., Gorer, R. and Newcombe, R. (1981). Carrier detection for haemophilia A in pregnancy. XIV Interntl. Congr. Wld. Fed. Haemophilia (Abstract)

15. Rodeck, C.H., Mibashan, R.S. and Campbell, S. (1981). Selective mid-trimester termination of congenitally abnormal twin by umbilical vascular air embolism. Prenatal Diagnosis (Submitted for publication)

16. Rodeck, C.H., Mibashan, R.S., Thumpston, J.K., Gorer, R. and Pietu, G. (1981). Prenatal diagnosis of Christmas disease (haemophilia B) Br. Med. J. (Submitted for publication)

Discussion

Dr. Tuddenham: In that clear and interesting presentation just one thing stood out for me - that we seem to have too few haemophiliac babies. Would you speculate on that?

Dr. Mibashan: A more detailed analysis will show that with 9 obligate carriers, one would expect the number of affected foetuses to be half, and in fact 4 were born. Those with a risk of carriership between 0.5 and unity numbered 24. Of those, the number who indeed are carriers might be of that order, with that resulting half-count, and in practice it was 7. There were 5 who came because they knew a relative whose life in the past had not been worth living, and their risk was on the low side. This is combining the effective criteria of pedigree and laboratory testing. It would statistically have been no more than one of those, perhaps, who might have been a real carrier, and it was not surprising that none of those produced a haemophiliac.

I think so long as a potential carrier is told that there is an 80-90 per cent chance that she is all right, but cannot be promised that, some of them, or their doctors will want to refer some of them in this imbalanced proportion.

Dr. Chediak: The possibility of a carrier was determined by the family tree?

Dr. Mibashan: By a combination of the family pedigree and laboratory testing, either at a recognised referring centre, and supplemented by testing in pregnancy, which incidentally appears valid, before fetoscopy.

Prof. Hoyer: In the Colonies we do not have anyone as skilled and as a result we have begun - back in 1978 and through to the present time - a prenatal diagnosis based not on pure blood samples aspirated from the foetus but rather on a mixture of foetal blood and amniotic fluid which is obtained by puncturing the chorionic plexus vessel and aspirating foetal blood at a 1:2 through a 1:10 dilution of amniotic fluid. Dr. Mibashan pointed out that this is probably unsatisfactory for coagulant assays, and we have not depended on it. However, the amniotic fluid does not have an effect on the immunologic assays for either coagulant antigen or Factor VIII related antigen. Our values for coagulant antigen measured in normal foetuses are very similar on blood that was eluted with amniotic fluid, and the values which you presented for direct puncture of the vessel.

With colleagues at Yale, who are fetoscopists of considerable experience we have been doing fetoscopies over this two-and-a-half year period to obtain prenatal diagnosis. Because we are not doing the direct foetal punctures, we cannot consider those families which are CRM positive, but the studies in a total of 33 women to the present time, some half of them carriers, 18 were positive carriers, or were to be considered strongly positive, and 8 women with a potential for being haemophiliac carriers but with negative assays.

In haemophilia 22 of the 33 were normal by combined coagulant antigen and Factor VIII related antigen measurements. Fifteen of those pregnancies have now gone to term verifying the normal state. In each of the cases in which haemophilia was diagnosed abortion was carried out and the diagnosis was again confirmed. We have no experience of non-identifiction. This is just to indicate that it is possible to also do prenatal diagnosis by means of aspiration of a mixture of foetal blood in amniotic fluid and that while it is very nice and comforting to have fetoscopists of such skill, if on your side of the ocean it does not happen, these families can still be counselled on proper information.

Dr. Mibashan: I hope that I did not give Dr. Hoyer or anyone present any impression other than that it is essential - admittedly in your series a very small proportion - something like 1:44 - but it is essential and extremely comforting to have the Factor VIII coagulant antigen assay in case of foetal dilution or of other activation or deterioration, and the risk is just dotting the i's and crossing the t's.

Orthopaedic Problems

18 Joint surgery in haemophilia

G. R. Houghton

This paper is an account of our experience of joint surgery in haemophilia at the Nuffield Orthopaedic Centre, Oxford, where patients were under the care of Professor Robert Duthie. The experience of other centres will be discussed particularly with reference to the more controversial methods of treatment.

The patient population under the care of the Haemophilia Centre is approximately 1000 which is one third of all haemophiliacs in the United Kingdom. Table 1 shows the distribution of these patients which have been admitted to the Nuffield Orthopaedic Centre for musculo-skeletal conditions between the years 1966-1979.

Table 1   Admissions 1966-1979

Disorder	Number of patients
Haemophilia A	603
Haemophilia B	45
von Willebrand's	7
TOTAL	655

The main reason for hospital admission was acute haemarthrosis and these patients suffered one or more bleeds as shown in the Table 2.

The Table closely reflects the incidence of chronic haemophilic arthropathy for which surgery is most often indicated. However, owing to the degree of development of reconstructive surgical techniques and their adaption to the anatomic variation of different joints, the rate of surgical intervention does not follow the incidence of haemarthrosis and chronic haemophilic arthropathy. For example, we have carried out 36 operations on the knee, 4 on the elbow and no less than 22 on the hip. All hip procedures were total joint replacements which reflects the known predictable good results of this procedure.

Table 2   Acute haemarthroses 1966-1979

Knee	363
Elbow	198
Ankle	110
Shoulder	28
Wrist	21
Hip	20
Hand	18
Foot	12
TOTAL	770

PRINCIPLES OF MANAGEMENT

A team approach to the surgical haemophilic patient is essential. As well as the orthopaedic and coagulation specialists, physiotherapists, occupational therapists, social workers, psychiatrists and orthotists as well as the ward staff should be fully trained and familiar in dealing with these patients.

The haematologist wishes to know:

1.   The circulating level of factor and the response to factor infusion.
2.   Whether antibodies are present.
3.   The nature and duration of proposed treatment.

These principles of coagulation control can only be carried out safely in Haemophilia Centres and with close liaison with the orthopaedic team. For any planned surgical treatment the total amount of factor required for the procedure and the entire post-operative period must be calculated and reserved for that particular patient.

Surgical Principles[1]

Standard surgical approaches and techniques are used. A pneumatic tourniquet will ensure a bloodless field and is only released after dressings have been applied. All dissection is carried out by electrocautery and meticulous haemostasis is achieved by diathermy coagulation. The wounds are closed by coaptation of tissue planes by continuous haemostatic polyglycolic acid (Dexon) sutures. Wounds are padded with a compression bandage and all adjacent joints immobilised in plaster of Paris splints. No drains, percutaneous pins or external fixation devices are used, in order to avoid the possible complication of pin track bleeding and infection. In general, definitive operations with predictable and good results are preferred to multiple staged surgical procedures.

With strict adherence to these principles factor consumption, hospital stay and complications have greatly diminished for each operation performed, and the complication rate is no greater than one would expect in a normal patient population.

LOWER LIMB JOINTS

The chief symptoms necessitating joint surgery are pain and stiffness and these indications are most frequently present in lower limb joints. Each joint will be considered in turn.

The Hip Joint

The hip joint is frequently affected by chronic haemophilic arthropathy although bleeds into the hip are not commonly diagnosed. Perhaps very few episodes of hip haemarthroses are sufficient to compromise the retinacular vessels and thus the blood supply to the femoral head[2]. Severe femoral capital destruction is not uncommon and does not respond to conservative management. Physiotherapy and analgesics temporarily alleviate symptoms but eventually surgery is indicated. Total hip replacement is the treatment of choice and the main indications are:

1.   Pain.
2.   Stiffness.
3.   Lesser degrees of 1 and 2 with other affected joints.

Table 3 shows our experience with total hip replacement. Extremes of age are not a contra-indication to the operation which is now a well established procedure with a low complication rate.

Table 3   Total hip replacement in 22 haemophilia patients

Procedure	No.	Factor needed	Duration of factor cover	In-patient stay
1. Cup arthroplasty	1	78 doses	70 days	85 days
2. McKee Farrar	4	55 doses	47 days	50 days
3. Charnley T.H.R.	17	Cases 1-10 43 doses		
			30 days	36 days
		Cases 11-17 61,000 units		

Age range 2-80.   Average 49.4 years.

The Charnely low friction arthroplasty is now routinely performed.   Removal of the greater trochanter as described by Charnley is avoided in haemophiliacs to diminish the bleeding surface of cancellous bone and thus haematoma formation.   Late problems with trochanteric wires and non-union are also eliminated.   Post-operatively the patient is immobilised in a plaster of Paris hip spica for 3 weeks and then gradually mobilised firstly in bed and then the hydrotherapy pool before walking on dry land.   Figure 1 shows the typical course of the patient undergoing total hip replacement. More recently, Epsicapron is added to the therapeutic regime to reduce factor requirement.   Our experience in normal patients shows that three weeks of plaster spica immobilisation does not prejudice the final range of movement in the hip.

There have been three major complications early on in the series. One patient underwent dislocation on the third post-operative day.   In this individual the plaster hip spica did not include the foot so that the affected lower extremity was able to rotate.   It is now our practice to include the entire operated lower extremity.   Another patient underwent a bleed into the rectus femoris muscle during the period of mobilisation, this was extremely painful but settled with Factor VIII replacement and a further period of immobilisation.   A further patient suffered a cardiac arrest during insertion of the femoral component.   A post-mortem was carried out and other than petechial brain haemorrhages secondary to anoxia, no cause for this complication was established. This patient unfortunately died on the fifth post-operative day.

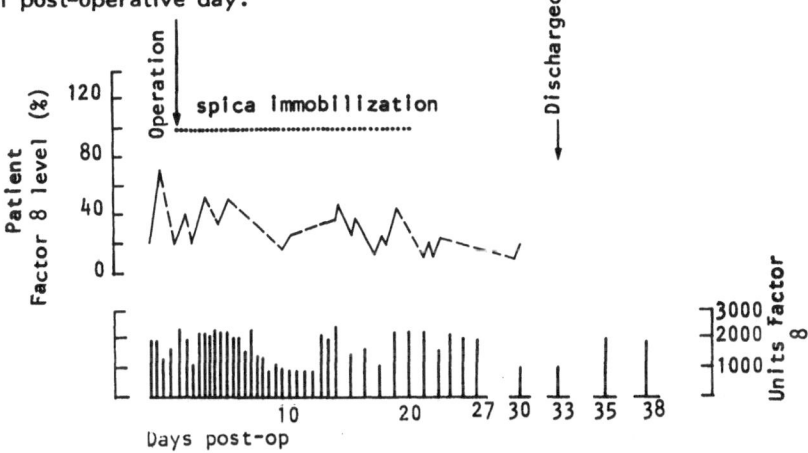

Figure 1   J.C. Total hip replacement   -   course

As well as severe haemophilic arthropathy of the hip, one patient presented with two pseudo-cysts in the buttock on the affected side. Prior to total hip replacement the cysts were excised and a routine total hip replacement was carried out 3 weeks later without complication.

Septic Arthritis

Unlike the other inflammatory arthropathies, haematogenous septic arthritis in haemophilia is very rare[3,4]. Our experience is one of one patient, a 32 year-old Factor VIII deficient haemophiliac with a high circulating titre of antibodies[5]. He developed a staphylococcal septic arthritis of the hip and was extremely toxic. Because of his high level of antibodies he was treated conservatively by aspiration and instillation of antibiotics on one occasion. High levels of parenteral antibiotics were administered and the hip was immobilised in a compression and plaster of Paris hip spica. There was complete resolution with this regime with a good painless range of motion.

The Knee Joint

The knee joint in haemophilia presents a major challenge to the attending physicians. With improving coagulation control our practice has been modified over recent years.

Acute Haemarthrosis

Acute haemarthrosis is usually managed conservatively by factor replacement, a Robert Jones compression bandage and plaster of Paris splint. Resolution is monitored by tape measurement. Static quadriceps drill is begun and immediately followed by dynamic exercises after resolution of the haemarthrosis, usually after 3 or 4 days. During the phase of mobilisation, the patient is supported by a bivalve splint, or if there is extreme quadriceps wasting and flexion contracture in a quadriceps enhancing orthosis.

Knee aspiration is now only rarely performed. The indications are as follows:

1. Unresolving acute haemarthrosis.
2. No synovitis, intra-articular adhesions, or arthropathy.
3. No antibodies.

Knee aspirations should be regarded as a <u>surgical</u> procedure in that it should be carried out under factor cover and full aseptic precautions in an operating theatre.

Sub-acute Haemarthrosis

Sub-acute haemarthrosis is a self-perpetuating pathological state consequent upon recurrent haemarthroses. The hypertrophic, hyperaemic synovium resulting from a haemarthrosis predisposes to further bleeding in the joint. The knee and elbow are particularly affected by this condition owing to the abundant synovium. The vicious cycle of events can be broken by effective non-operative treatment. Factor replacement and immobilisation of the knee joint in a padded plaster splint for a period of 3-4 weeks will usually result in a gradual resolution of the swelling. Isometric quadriceps exercises are carried out during this period to prevent muscle atrophy which may delay the mobilisation period and which may be responsible for allowing the condition to recur in some individuals.

If after 3 or 4 weeks the swelling and thickening has resolved, the patient is mobilised gradually under factor cover. Hydrotherapy is instituted to give additional support during the weight bearing period and regain useful range of motion in a further 3 weeks.

If resolution does not take place in a further 4 weeks, the patient may undergo a further 3 week period of immobilisation with factor cover. The majority of patients will respond to this regime.

Occasionally the vicious cycle cannot be broken and the patient retains a boggy synovial thickening with recurrent haemarthrosis. In these circumstances synovectomy may be necessary as a haemostatic procedure[6-8]. The value of synovectomy is not yet proven, but its rationale is based on the fact that the synovium is intimately involved in the eventual destruction of the articular surface and the progressive contracture and deformation of the knee joint. The removal of the hypertrophic hyperaemic synovium with the elevated levels of cathepsin D should reduce the risk of further haemorrhage into the joint and arrest the destruction of articular cartilage. However, synovectomy is contra-indicated in a patient with high levels of antibody or in the very young patient with a chronically swollen knee. In the latter case, the consequences for the nutrition of articular cartilage are not known. These patients can be immobilised in an ischial bearing caliper with knee support for up to 6 months with resolution of the synovial hypertrophy and recurrent bleeds. We have carried out 7 synovectomies and all have regained an excellent range of motion with marked decrease in subsequent frequency in large intra-articular bleeds. However, 2 patients have developed small haemorrhages outside the newly formed synovial lining which was very painful. A third patient has undergone manipulation under anaesthetic at 3 weeks post-operatively. There have recently been encouraging reports of chemical and radio-active synovectomies from Sweden and France. The long-term results from these procedures, however, are not known, and we prefer a surgical approach.

Chronic Haemophilic Arthropathy

Despite the correct management of acute and sub-acute haemarthroses, chronic haemophilic arthropathy of the knee is still common. Surgery still plays a relatively minor role in its treatment and is not considered before exhausting the full repertoire of conservative management. Treatment regimes fall into four categories:

1. Physiotherapy.
2. Orthotics.
3. Corrective devices.
4. Reconstructive surgery.

1. Physiotherapy

The main aim of physiotherapy to the knee is to maintain good quadricepts muscle power. Knowing that exercise may increase the level of circulating Factor VIII, physiotherapy may be regarded as a form of prophylactic treatment[9]. Both static and dynamic exercises are carried out to promote mobile and stable joints. However, muscle power alone will not overcome dense intra-articular adhesions and quadriceps power will be compromised by a fixed flexion deformity owing to mechanical influences. In the presence of these problems other methods are employed while physiotherapy continues.

2.   Orthotics

Lightweight plastic splints and calipers are used extensively for the protection and support of the knee joint following repeated haemarthroses. It is important to prevent muscle atrophy while the affected joint is protected by any form of external splintage. In the presence of a fixed flexion deformity of 20° or less, passive and dynamic quadriceps exercises can be carried out in an open fronted orthoplast splint. Its use is not confined to patients with chronic haemophilic arthropathy but may be used for correcting flexion deformities following acute haemarthroses or those secondary to soft tissue bleeds in the hamstrings and calf muscles.

3.   Corrective appliances: reverse dynamic slings

This technique has been developed over the last 10 years and is now the method of choice for the correction of fixed flexion contractures of the knee. It has the advantage that quadriceps muscle power and tone are improved and enables physiotherapy to be carried out at the same time. Movement of the knee restored by the technique reduces the tendency to intra-articular adhesion formation and aids the nutrition of articular cartilage.

The method is described elsewhere[10]. A prospective study of this technique of reverse dynamic slings comparing the results with serial plaster casts has shown the slings to be significantly superior. Both groups had severe fixed flexion deformities at the knee, present for a mean duration of 3 years. The mean age of the cast patients was 19.5 years and the mean age of the sling patients was 17.5 years. In the patients with reverse dynamic slings, the flexion contracture was reduced by an average of 34.6° compared with 9.4° in the serial plaster group. The mean treatment time was significantly reduced in the dynamic sling group (14 days) when compared with serial cast group (30 days).

The majority of patients in each group have increased their range of motion. There was no correlation between the duration of fixed flexion contracture and the length of time required to reach the final correction in each group. The method is therefore suitable for the treatment of long standing deformity. None of the patients that have been treated in this way has had any complications and factor replacement has not been routine.

4. Reconstructive surgery

Table 4 lists the surgical procedures formed in the knee from 1966-1979.

Table 4   Surgical procedures performed in the knee (1966-1979)

Procedure	Number of patients
Evacuation of haematoma	4
Patellectomy	4
Removal of exostosis	1
Manipulation under anaesthetic	3
Meniscectomy	7
Synovectomy	7
Arthrodesis	11
TOTAL	37

Evacuation of haematoma was carried out in the late 1960's in 4 patients. They fell into the group of patients which we now recognise as having sub-acute haemarthrosis. These patients have been presented, several days or weeks after the initial haemarthrosis, with hot, swollen and painful knees. Palpation of the joint content revealed a doughy semi-solid knee; evidence that the haemarthrosis had clotted. The aetiology and treatment of this state has already been discussed and this procedure is no longer performed.

Patellectomy has been carried out on 4 patients. Recurrent pain and swelling have been the presenting symptoms. In one patient the swelling had been proven to be synovial fluid by aspiration. All the patients had painful retropatellar crepitus with a restricted range of motion. There was radiological evidence of patello femoral arthritis with variable involvement of the tibio femoral component of the knee joint. The operation is carried out by a small medial para-patellar incision with careful dissection of the attachment of the quadriceps and patellar tendon fibres from the patella. The defect is closed in layer with opposing Dexon sutures and the leg supported in a plaster of Paris cylinder for 3 weeks. Thereafter the patient is mobilised under factor cover. The results following this procedure have been variable; one patient being rendered symptom free with a range of motion of 5-90°. One patient has had persistent pain and haemarthrosis with a range of movement of 0-68°. A further patient was slow to mobilise and required manipulation under anaesthetic. Two of the patients underwent simultaneous synovectomy. It would seem that a concomitant synovectomy in a patient having patellectomy and a longer period of immobilisation gives rise to a dry stiff joint and in this type of joint small isolated haemarthroses with stiffness frequently occur.

One patient has required the removal of a loose body in his knee which was giving rise to haemarthrosis and locking. There was complete relief of his symptoms.

Manipulation under anaesthetic is of value in the post-operative phase following patellectomy or synovectomy to break down intra-articular adhesions under factor cover.

The haemophilic patient's knee is subject to internal derangement in the same way as a normal persons would be. Seven medical meniscectomies have been carried out on 6 patients in the last 13 years. Four of the patients had Factor VIII deficiency and 2 Factor IX deficiency. One patient had bilateral procedures. Three of the patients had a significant rotational injury to the knee and in 4 knees symptoms arose spontaneously. The symptoms have included intermittent pain, swelling, locking and instability.

Four of the patients had medial joint line tenderness and one had a mechanical block to extension. None of the patients had a significant haemophilic arthropathy at the time of surgery, although one patient required a patellectomy and synovectomy 2 years later. One of the patients with Christmas disease had an arthroscopy prior to arthrotomy. On this occasion a bucket handle lesion could be easily identified and removed. Total meniscectomy was carried out on 6 occasions and in one patient the bucket handle section only was removed. The combined use of the arthroscope and the current thoughts on the value of minimal procedures may allow a more selective policy for meniscectomy in the future[11]. The results in all cases were excellent.

Arthrodesis Of The Knee

When a painful fixed flexion contracture of the knee becomes permanent and functionally disabling, arthrodesis has proved to be a valuable procedure. Eleven arthrodeses have been carried out over an 11 year period. Pain was the main indication in all cases with additonal indications of deformity, instability and recurrent haemarthroses. The average range of motion of the affected joint was 31° compared with 92° on the unaffected side.

The technique involves full haemostatic control. An average of 28,000 units of Factor VIII was required for each arthrodesis. The following steps are carried out via a median para-patellar incision:

1. Excision of the articular surfaces of the patella, femur and tibia.
2. Internal fixation with compression using crossed threaded cancellous screws.
3. The knee is arthrodesed in between 10 and 30° of flexion depending upon co-existent hip or ankle deformity.

Complications of the procedure include 3 cases of delayed union of 7, 11 and 12 months respectively. One haematoma and one wound infection. The 2 latter complications settled with conservative therapy.

Post-operatively the leg is protected in a long leg plaster of Paris cast, which is changed at 2 weeks when the sutures are removed. Isometric quadriceps exercises are commenced early and maintained until the supportive cast is removed, when there is radiological union at the site of the arthrodesis.

Knee arthrodesis is a successful definitive procedure in the haemophilic patient despite the not uncommon complication of poor wound healing and superficial infection. However, these complications did not require further surgical intervention. The procedure renders the haemophiliac knee pain-free and thereby avoids the use of further factor and all its attendant dangers.

Total Knee Arthroplasty

Over the last 5 years, reports of total knee replacement in the haemophiliac have been appearing in the literature[6,7,8,13,14]. The knee is much more frequently affected by the haemophilic arthropathy than the hip. However, the good results are seen commonly in total hip replacement but not following arthroplasty of the knee. Total hip arthroplasty is a predictably successful procedure in the haemophilic patient, whereas total knee arthroplasty definitely is not[12].

The procedure has been advocated for patients with bilateral disease, or in limbs with ipsilateral hip or ankle disease[7]. The main symptoms have been secondary to destructive disease of the joint. The procedure is contra-indicated for the small deformed contracted joint with flexion, valgus and rotational deformities. It is also contra-indicated in patients with marked contractural fibrosis and wasting of the quadriceps[6]. Unfortunately it is just these knees which are the most painful and have the least range of movement.

Synovectomy has been carried out simultaneously by most authors[7,13,14]. The majority of patients have been in their 3rd, 4th and 5th decades. The operation is definitely contra-indicated in the haemophiliac in his 1st and 2nd decades. The older haemophilic patient seems to require less factor during the period of surgery than in the post-operative phase when compared with synovectomy in the younger patient. It has been suggested that the older haemophilic patient, like his counterpart with rheumatoid arthritis, transmits relatively little load through the knee joint[7].

The main advantage to be gained from total knee arthroplasty would appear to be relief of pain[7,8,15]. The restoration of joint movement is of secondary consequence and variable in its achievement. The functional gain outweighs any loss of mobility. Any reduction of the incidence of haemarthrosis will have to be evaluated in the context of the individual patient and not advocated as an indication for the technique of total knee arthroplasty. We would not, at the present time, advocate total knee replacement in the adolescent early onset chronic haemophilic arthropathy. We would also advise caution in using this procedure even in the older haemophilic patient. The majority of reports have come from small series, up to 8 patients, with a short follow-up.

The only comparable, but larger group of patients, which have been critically studied following total knee arthroplasty, using both hinged and unconstrained implants are patients with juvenile chronic polyarthritis (Still's disease). Arden reported a series with 37 total joint replacements of the knee in 26 polyarthritic patients[16]. The average age of the patients was 25 years with a follow-up from 1-9 years, averaging 4 years only. Only 54% of patients had an excellent to good result with a 46% failure rate. Of the failures, 7 were due to infection, 8 due to stiffness and 2 due to loosening. There was a 19% infection rate.

Among the reported cases of total knee replacement, several authors had minor or no complications[6,8,13,14]. However, in the comparatively large series by McCollough of 10 arthroplasties in 8 patients, the following complications were noted[7]: 3 haemarthroses, one late loosening of the tibial component, and one infection. We believe that this complication rate is unacceptable in a group of patients who are already exposed to lethal complications as a result of the natural history and treatment of this disease.

The Ankle Joint

The ankle joint is a common site for acute haemarthroses and accordingly chronic haemophilic arthropathy is frequently seen. Joint disease is further exacerbated by the frequency of calf haematomata leading to contractures and equinus ankle deformity. If equinus deformity is absent, pain in the ankle will usually respond to orthotic support in the form of a caliper, or now the much preferred Yates plastic splint.

Equinus deformity with contracted calf muscles will not respond to stretching exercises or any other conservative procedure. The only alternative to heel raises and modified footwear is surgery.

Elongation of the tendo Achilles has been carried out in 14 cases and only if there is no radiological evidence of significant haemophiliac arthropathy in the ankle joint. A standard medial approach is used with a Z plasty tendon elongation. A posterior capsulectomy of the ankle joint is usually carried out. This ensures a good correction of the deformity and also permits a visual appraisal of the ankle joint.

Chronic haemophilic arthropathy of the ankle joint with pain and stiffness can be managed satisfactorily with below knee calipers, but arthrodesis which avoids external orthoses is now often advised. The technique is the Royal Air Force method of joint excision and fibular onlay grafting[17]. This method avoids percutaneous pins of the compression technique most commonly used in normal patients. In a series of 9 patients, all ankles were solidly fused in less than 6 months and the only complications were 2 cases of delayed wound healing[12]. As in knee arthrodeses no secondary surgical procedures were required.

Although total ankle prostheses are available, the effect of this procedure is little more than an arthrodesis with the additional risks of infection and loosening. There is no place for total ankle replacement in haemophilia.

Rigid equinus deformity in the mid foot region is not uncommon in haemophilia and is rarely passively correctable. The only alternative to the wearing of surgical boots is a <u>wedge tarsectomy</u> and this has been carried out in 6 patients, 2 of which had a simultaneous elongation of the tendo Achilles. There has been one serious complication of this operation with sloughing of the skin of the dorsum of the foot, which required skin grafting and took 6 weeks to heal.

UPPER LIMB JOINTS

Elective joint surgery in the upper limb is rarely performed, as chronic haemophilic arthropathy is generally less severe than in the weight bearing joints of the lower limb, which are under greater stress.

No procedures have been carried out on the shoulder joint.

Elbow contractures frequently occur and usually respond to dynamic slings similar to the arrangement as described in the knee joint. On 3 occasions radial head excision and synovectomy has been carried out for stiff painful elbow joints. The procedure is followed by a gratifying result with pain relief and an improved range of movement in every case.

Elbow deformity may predispose to ulnar neuritis and transposition of the nerve has been carried out with 2 patients, with complete resolution of symptoms.

CONCLUSIONS

Unlike joint surgery in degenerative disease, the haemophilic patient has the additional disadvantage of a coagulation disorder which may compromise the surgical result or even the patient's life[18]. The decision to perform surgery should not be taken lightly. Only well tried methods should be advised and not new or experimental procedures, which have not been proved in non-haemophilic patients.

The management of haemophilic arthopathy makes many demands on the skill and patience of the doctors concerned. It is hoped that the progression of home therapy and better education of the patient will reduce the problems which have to be dealt with in the future.

REFERENCES

1. Duthie, R.B., Mathews, J.M, Rizza, C.R. and Steel, W.M. (1972). The management of musculo-skeletal problems in the haemophilias. (Oxford: Blackwell Scientific Publications)

2. Kemp, H.B.S. (1965). Some observations on Perthes' Disease. J. Bone Joint Surg., 47B, 193

3. Goldenberg, D.L., Brandt, K.D., Cohen, A.S. and Cathcart, E.S. (1975). Treatment of septic arthritis. Arthr. Rheum., 18, 83

4. Kellgren, J.H., Ball, J., Fairbrother, R.W. and Barnes, K.L. (1958). Suppurative arthritis complicating rheumatoid arthritis. Br. Med. J., 1, 1193

5. Houghton, G.R. (1977). Septic arthritis of the hip in a haemophiliac. Clin. Orthroped., 129, 223

6. Arnold, W.D. and Hilgartner, M.W. (1977). Haemophiliac arthropathy. J. Bone Joint Surg., 59A, 287

7. McCollough, N.C., Enis, J.E., Lovitt, J., Lian, E.C., Niemann, K.N.W. and Loughlin, E.C. (1979). Synovectomy or total replacement of the knee in haemophilia. J. Bone Joint Surg., 61A, 69

8. Post, M. and Teifer, M.C. (1975). Surgery in haemophilic patients. J. Bone Joint Surg., 57A, 1136

9. Rizza, C.R. (1961). Effect of exercise on the level of antihaemophilic globulin in human blood. J. Physiol., 156, 128

10. Stein, H. and Dickson, R.A. (1975). Reversed dynamic slings for knee flexion contractures in the haemophiliac. J. Bone Joint Surg., 57A, 282

11. Goodfellow, J.W. (1980). He who hesitates is saved. Editorial. J. Bone Joint Surg., 62B, 1

12. Houghton, G.R. and Dickson, R.A. (1978). Lower limb arthrodeses in haemophilia. J. Bone Joint Surg., 60B, 143

13. London, J.T., Kattlove, H., Louie, J.S. and Forster, G.L. (1977). Synovectomy and total joint arthroplasty for recurrent haemarthrosis in the arthropathic joint in haemophilia. Arthr. Rheum., 20, 8

14. Marmor, L. (1977). Total knee replacement in haemophilia. Clin. Orthoped., 125, 192

15. Hilgartner, M.W. (1973). Pathogenesis of joint changes in haemophilia. In: McCollough, N.C. (ed.) Comprehensive Management of Musculo-Skeletal Disorders in Haemophilia, p. 33. (Washington: National Academy of Sciences)

16. Arden, G.P. (1978). Total joint replacement. In: Arden, G.P. and Ansell, B.M. (eds.) Surgical Management of Chronic Juvenile Polyarthritis, p. 146. (Academic Press, London: Grune and Stratton, New York)

17. Adams, J.C. (1948). Arthrodesis of the ankle joint. J. Bone Joint Surg., 30B, 506

18. Houghton, G.R. and Duthie, R.B. (1979). Orthopaedic problems in haemophilia. Clin. Orthoped., 138, 197

Discussion

<u>Anonymous</u>:   Would you say some more about the use of the arthroscope, and what you feel the indications are for this.

<u>Mr. Houghton</u>:   It is important to use an arthroscope if a patient has an internal derangement of the knee joint, such as a meniscectomy or a loose body, and the surgeon wants to see what it is that is causing the problem.   I do not think otherwise it has a place in patients with chronic haemophilic arthropathy.   If a synovial biopsy is to be taken for any reason, then of course it is very useful for that, and also to assess the inside of the joint.   We have only carried out one arthroscopy, which was very useful in that particular patient, but we do not do it routinely.

Index

235